Immunology Investigations:

A Laboratory Manual

Loreli A. Batina, MS

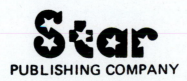

Star
PUBLISHING COMPANY

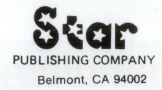

Star
PUBLISHING COMPANY
Belmont, CA 94002

Star Publishing Company
P.O. Box 68
Belmont, CA 94002-0068

Managing Editor: Stuart A. Hoffman
Consulting Editor: Dr. Susan G. Kelley

ISBN: 0-89863-176-9   Printed in Korea   0987654321   97 98 99

Table of Contents

Section 3   Advanced Exercises in Immunology 121

Appendices

Introduction

Immunology is a field which has drawn keen interest in recent years due in part to the great advances made possible by new techniques in molecular biology, and to the increased public awareness of issues involving the AIDS crisis, cancer, organ transplants, and other formidable medical problems. The objective of this manual is to introduce students to this exciting field in a laboratory setting, and to provide them with experience in many of the methods currently used in clinical and research immunology.

This manual presents a wide variety of exercises suitable for use at the advanced undergraduate level. It is not meant to cover all aspects of immunology, but to serve as a laboratory supplement to a lecture course and textbook in immunology. The manual includes more exercises than can be carried out in a single semester, allowing the instructor to choose those that are of greatest interest or are the most practical in the given teaching facilities. For example, a few exercises require specialized equipment or reagents like the scintillation counter and radioisotope used in exercise 23, and may not be feasible for all institutions. Most exercises do not require unusual equipment. The exercises themselves range from simple, three-hour procedures to fairly challenging exercises that require more than one laboratory period. Either the rabbit immunization exercise or the monoclonal antibody exercise could be used as a semester-long project.

The exercises have been developed over a period of years at Washington State University, and each has been performed successfully by students in the classroom–laboratory. In fact, the subjects for all photographs in this manual were provided by students. While some of the photography may not be perfect, it is the author's aim to show that students may obtain good results from these exercises. The procedures given have also been designed for flexibility, because not every instructor will have the same equipment, budget, and class size. A separate instructor's guide is available that includes additional information for the instructor, including how to set up the exercises; various alternatives to the procedures, reagents, organisms or equipment used and how to implement the changes;

where alternative materials can be obtained; and common student errors that occur for each procedure.

The manual has three sections based on subject matter and most logical use of reagents and equipment. Each exercise begins with an introduction for the student, followed by a materials list, experimental procedure, study questions, and reading list. Particular attention has been paid to safety issues and sensitivity to student concerns towards use of experimental animals. The manual begins with basic up-to-date safety rules for the classroom and includes an appendix dealing specifically with safety and the use of laboratory animals. In addition, each exercise includes a short list of safety precautions specific to the procedure, where warranted.

It is hoped that through this manual students will gain experience in many immunological techniques used in laboratories, as well as in important laboratory skills that they may use in their future careers.

Acknowledgments

This manual would not have been possible without the input of the many W. S. U. students I have taught. Their enthusiasm and willingness to "go the extra mile" has been the inspiration for this project. I am particularily grateful to the graduate teaching assistants who have provided much insight over the years; to Dr. Nancy S. Magnuson, who provided encouragement as I experimented with the course; and to my husband, Ray, and daughter, Julia, who were very patient during all my hours of typing.

⚠ *Laboratory Safety*

The laboratory exercises included in this manual may be hazardous if the materials or equipment are handled improperly or if procedures are conducted incorrectly. Before performing any exercise or experiment in this text, you must be trained and instructed in the proper techniques for the procedures, equipment, and materials involved. If you have not been so instructed, do not perform the exercise or experiment until you have been trained and instructed.

Safety precautions are necessary when you are working with chemicals, microbiological cultures, glassware, hot water baths, animals, sharp instruments, and other equipment, materials, or procedures in this course. Your school has set regulations regarding safety procedures that your instructor will explain to you.

Read the appropriate sections of this laboratory manual before the laboratory session so that you will know what is to be done and the basic principles involved.

Should you have any problems or questions about equipment, chemicals, materials, microbiological cultures or media, or procedures, ask your instructor for help. If you have any questions at all about what to do or not to do, stop and do not proceed until you are fully aware and knowledgeable about the procedure you are doing.

The experiments and procedures in this text are only to be carried out under the supervision of a trained instructor. Do not perform any laboratory experiment or procedure in the absence of such supervision.

The following safety precautions should be taken seriously and practiced every lab period. There will be additional safety information given with each exercise and from your instructor to alert you to any specific hazards.

Chemical, physical, and biological hazards are a reality of any laboratory work. Part of your training as a scientist is becoming aware of and learning to work safely with these hazards. Read appendix 5 before starting any laboratory session.

1. Upon entering the laboratory, place your books, bag, coat, and other items in the areas provided at the side of the room. Put on your lab coat, clean your bench top by wiping with disinfectant, and wash your hands. This lab manual and a lab notebook should be the only personal items on or near your bench.

2. Eating, drinking, smoking, taking medicine, applying cosmetics, licking labels, storing food, or anything else involving putting something in your mouth is not allowed in the laboratory.

3. Mouth pipetting is strictly forbidden.

4. Long hair should be tied back. Turn off your bunsen burner if you are not actually using it.

5. Gloves and safety goggles should be worn when working with human blood or body fluids, or anytime a procedure has the potential for aerosolization. Avoid contact with any human blood or body fluids other than your own.

6. Do *not* re-cap syringes, or lay them on the lab bench. If you must set a syringe aside for a moment, place it inside a sterile tube in a rack.

7. Perform only specifically assigned exercises. Performance of unauthorized experiments is strictly forbidden.

8. Notify the instructor of *any* spill, cut, burn, or accident.

9. Never dispose of any chemical down the sink drain. Set all media, cultures, and reagents in the designated discard area when finished. If appropriate discard

bins and disinfectant containers are not available, see your instructor.

10. If a spill of possibly infectious materials occurs, first remove your lab coat if it has been spilled on. Cover the spill with paper towels and flood with 5% chlorox. Allow the chlorox to contact the spilled material for at least 20 minutes. Do not touch broken glass with your hands. Use a broom and dustpan to clean up the mess and place in an autoclavable container. Wash your hands when finished.

11. Wash your hands with antiseptic soap any time you think you might have contaminated them, if you leave the laboratory, and at the conclusion of the laboratory session.

12. Dispose of all laboratory materials only in the manner prescribed. In particular, place broken glass and syringe needles only in the containers designed for that purpose, and never in the trash.

13. Before leaving the laboratory, clean up and disinfect your bench; remove your lab coat, then wash your hands. The lab coats are to remain in the laboratory.

Section 1

Introduction to the Immune System

Immunity is the ability of the body to resist disease. Immune responses are carried out by an array of molecular substances and immune cells that circulate throughout the blood and lymphatic systems. The body has two levels of immunity; **innate immunity** which can fight infection even at the very first encounter with a pathogen, and **acquired immunity**, which is highly effective but develops only after the pathogen has already been "seen" and "memorized".

Acquired immunity is mediated by specific immune cells called **lymphocytes** and is the type of immunity that is most often manipulated to prevent disease. For example, vaccination brings about acquired immunity. Acquired immunity can be further divided into **humoral immunity** and **cellular immunity**. Humoral immunity involves the antibody proteins produced in response to infection or vaccination. These proteins are manufactured by B cell lymphocytes. Cellular immunity involves activities mainly carried out by the T cell lymphocytes that cause graft rejection, fight cancer, and attack certain intracellular pathogens like viruses and the bacterium that causes tuberculosis.

The first section of this manual is designed to introduce you to the components and activities of the immune system.

Cells and Organs of the Immune System

The immune system protects the body both from outward invaders like viruses, bacteria, fungi, and parasites, and from inner threats like cancer. To carry out these functions, the immune system must be able to distinguish "foreign" materials (**antigens**) from the body's own components, and also control the magnitude of the immune response. The complex array of activities occurring during an immune response are orchestrated by a variety of immune cells. These cells are dispersed throughout the blood and tissues, but tend to concentrate in the **lymphoid organs** (fig. 1.1).

The lymphoid organs consist of **primary lymphoid organs**, in which the immune cells develop, and **secondary lymphoid organs**, in which mature immune cells carry out their functions. A network of lymphatic vessels allows circulation of the immune cells between the tissues, the bloodstream, and the lymphoid organs. In this exercise you will be observing some of the lymphoid organs in the mouse (fig. 1.2).

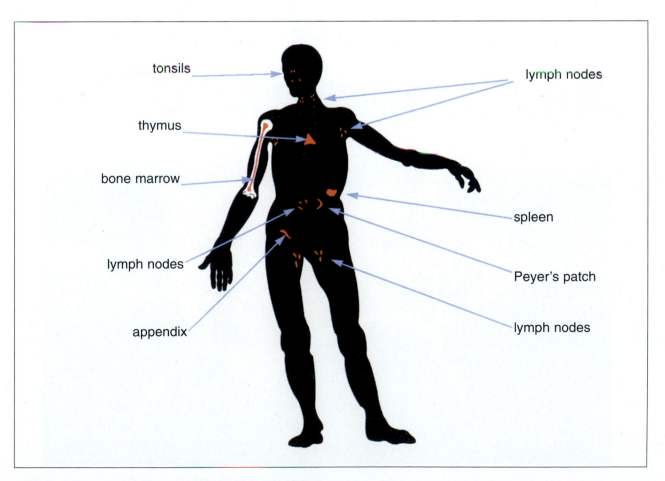

tonsils

lymph nodes

thymus

bone marrow

spleen

lymph nodes

Peyer's patch

appendix

lymph nodes

Figure 1.1   Location of the lymphoid organs in humans

A. Primary Lymphoid Organs— organs in which immune cells develop.

1. *Bone marrow*: site of the development of all the blood cells, including immune cells. The process of blood cell development is called **hemopoesis**. Blood cells in various stages of development can be found in the red marrow.

2. *Thymus*: organ in which the T-lymphocyte immune cells develop. The thymus is a greyish organ with two lobes. It lies directly above the heart. The thymus consists of an outer layer called the cortex that contains densely packed immature lymphocytes, and an inner area called the medulla that contains more loosely packed mature lymphocytes and epithelial cells (fig. 1.3A).

B. Secondary Lymphoid Organs— organs in which mature immune cells carry out their functions.

1. *Spleen*: an encapsulated organ which consists of networks of blood and lymphatic vessels and two main types of tissue; **red pulp** and **white pulp**. The red pulp consists mostly of erythrocytes, while the white pulp consists of areas rich in white blood cells (fig. 1.3B). The spleen is a red, flat, finger-like organ found directly under the stomach on the left side.

2. *Lymph Nodes*: small encapsulated organs located at strategic sites along the body's network of blood vessels and lymphatic vessels. They may be found embedded in the connective tissue in the neck area, the armpits and groin, and in the mesenteric membrane of the intestines. The lymph nodes contain

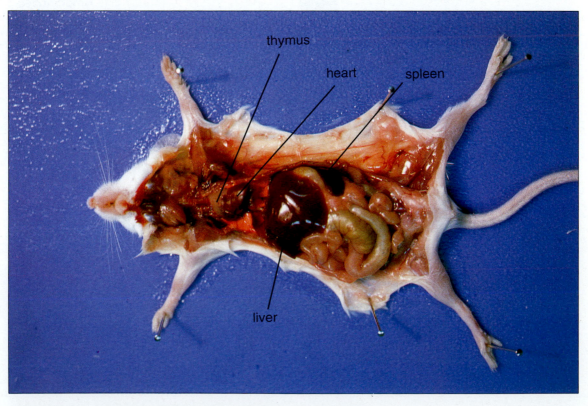

Figure 1.2   Location of the lymphoid organs in the mouse

primary follicles, which are areas where immune cells aggregate and respond to antigen (fig. 1.3C).

3. *Mucosal Associated Lymphoid Tissue* (*MALT*): a general term for the unencapsulated lymphoid tissues found in association with submucosal areas of the respiratory, gastrointestinal, and genitourinary tracts. It includes the **tonsils** and the **Peyer's patches** of the intestines.

C.   Cells of the Immune System

The blood contains **erythrocytes** (red blood cells or "RBCs"), **leukocytes** (white blood cells or "WBCs"), and **platelets** suspended in a liquid called plasma (fig. 1.4). The basic properties and functions of the blood cells are listed in table 1.2. Erythrocytes are formed in the bone marrow and, in mammals, extrude their nuclei before entering the circulation. The leukocytes remain nucleated and consist of two major types: granular and agranular. The granular **leukocytes**, **neutrophils**, **basophils**, and **eosinophils**, have cytoplasmic granules which contain enzymes involved in the destruction of foreign material in the body. The agranular leukocytes include the **monocytes** and **lymphocytes**. Lymphocytes are further subdivided into groups including B-cells and T-cells. The platelets are very small non-nucleated particles formed by the break-up of bone marrow megakaryocytes. They are often seen in clusters in a blood smear.

There are many human diseases which cause variations in the numbers or types of blood cells. For example, many infectious diseases exhibit an increased lymphocyte or neutrophil count, and leukemias usually cause the appearance of large numbers of both mature and immature cells not normally found in the peripheral blood.

For this exercise you will examine the variety of cells found in the peripheral blood and lymphoid organs. The histology and function of these organs will be discussed, and the lymphoid organs of the mouse will be located. You will also prepare smears of peripheral blood. These smears will be

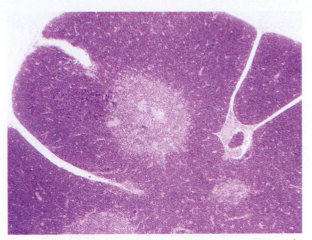

A.   The thymus: note the dense outer cortex and the more loosely packed inner medulla.

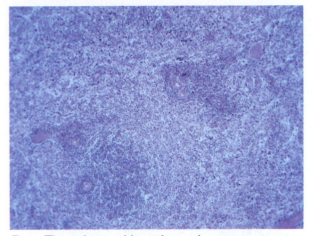

B.   The spleen: white pulp can be seen as areas of white blood cells usually surrounding a blood vessel.

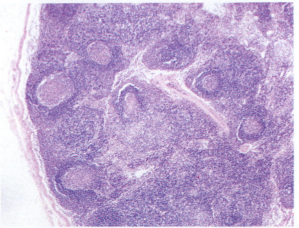

C.   A lymph node: note the round-shaped follicles within the organ.

Figure 1.3   Tissue cross-sections of lymphoid organs. The white blood cells stain purple.

stained with Wright's stain and examined micro-scopically for cell content.

Materials:

- [ ] mouse
- [ ] mouse jar with anesthetic and cotton balls
- [ ] dissecting board, pins, scissors, and forceps
- [ ] 70% ethanol in a squirt bottle
- [ ] sterile lancet
- [ ] small bottle of 70% ethanol or an alcohol swab
- [ ] cotton balls
- [ ] finger-tip bandage
- [ ] 5 glass microscope slides
- [ ] Wright's stain and Wright's buffer, or Volu-Sol™ Stat stain

Procedure:

A. Dissection of Mouse

1. Euthanize a mouse by placing it in a jar or coffee can which contains a couple of cotton balls soaked in chloroform. Close the jar tightly for 5 minutes.

2. Wet down the euthanized mouse with 70% ethanol. Pin down the four feet on a dissecting board with steel pins. Pull up the skin of the abdomen with the forceps and cut through the abdomen longitudinally with the scissors. Cut and fold back the skin and muscles of the abdomen to expose the internal organs. Locate the thymus, spleen, and some lymph nodes, then dispose of the mouse carcass in the container designated for that purpose.

B. Preparation of Peripheral Blood Smear

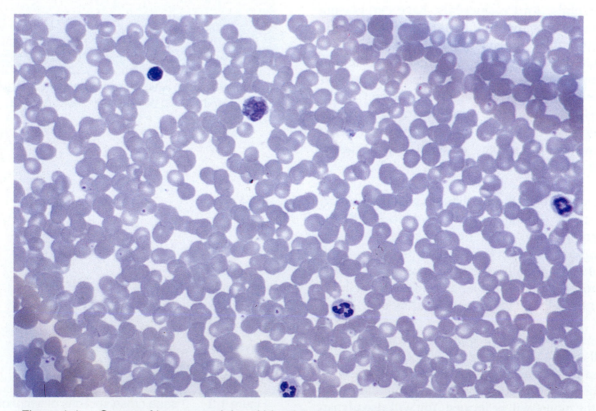

Figure 1.4   Smear of human peripheral blood stained with Wright's stain. Many erythrocytes can be seen, and also a lymphocyte, a monocyte, and neutrophils.

⚠ *Safety Tips:*
1.   **Avoid breathing anesthetic vapors.**
2.   **Be careful not to let ethanol drip down onto your hand when flaming dissection tools, and do not place hot dissection tools directly into the ethanol or touch the ethanol-doused mouse.**
3.   **If an ethanol fire does occur, don't panic or use water, but simply smother the fire with a beaker or towel.**
4.   **Prick your own finger and handle only your own blood smear. Do not exchange lancets.**
5.   **All sharp objects, including pins and lancets, are to be disposed of in a biohazard container. Under no circumstances are they to be thrown in the trash cans.**
6.   **Wright's stain is a flammable poison. Keep it away from sparks or flames. The vapor is harmful if inhaled.**

1.   Clean the microscope slides with ethanol and an appropriate lens-cleaning tissue.

2.   Have a sterile lancet and a clean, dry cotton ball ready. Clean your left "ring" finger tip with an alcohol-soaked cotton ball and let it air dry.

3.   Puncture your finger with the lancet, trying to strike at the side of the finger tip to avoid the calloused skin in the center.

4.   Discard the first drop of blood by wiping it away with the cotton ball.

5.   Place a drop of blood on the left end of each of four clean slides. When preparing a peripheral blood smear it is essential that the drop of blood be drawn out to a feather-thin edge. This allows you to find an area of the smear under the microscope where the cells are only one layer thick and easily visible for identification and counting. It may be neces-

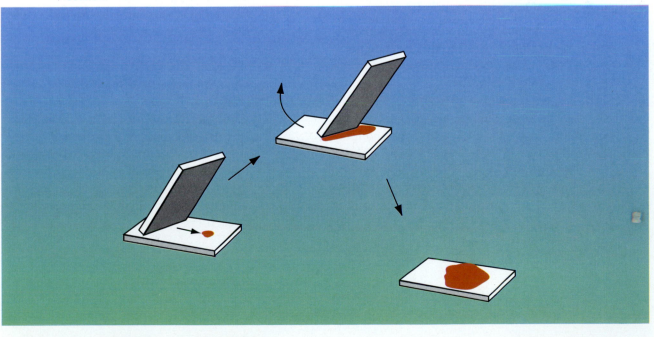

Figure 1.5   Preparation of a Blood Smear

sary to practice a few times before a good smear is obtained (fig. 1.5).

6. Place the slide on a firm surface and hold down with your left hand. Hold a second "spreader" slide in the right hand over the lower slide, and at an angle of 45° move this slide from right to left across the lower slide until the edge of the spreader slide comes in contact with the drop of blood. As soon as the drop of blood is contacted it will flow along the bottom edge of the spreader slide. With one quick, smooth motion, push the spreader back from left to right, pulling the blood behind it. Do not push the blood in front of the spreader slide or pull the slide over the smear twice. Repeat with the other three slides if necessary.

7. Let the smears air dry, and then stain with Wright's stain (part C), or Stat stain (part D).

C.   Wright's Stain Procedure

1. Obtain dropper bottles of Wright's stain and Wright's buffer.

2. Cover the smears with Wright's stain for 2 to 3 minutes. During this time *do not let the slides dry out*. Continue adding more stain if necessary.

3. Add an approximately equal amount of buffer to the slide and allow to stand for 3 minutes. Again, *do not* let the slides dry out but keep adding buffer as needed. Blow gently across the slide every few minutes to mix the solutions.

4. Gently rinse the slide by continual washing with water from one end until

the water runs clear. *Do not* simply pour off the stain as this will leave precipitated stain on the slide.

5. Allow the smears to air dry.

6. Examine the peripheral blood smears. Identify cell types and perform a differential count: count a total of 100 white blood cells, recording the numbers of each type observed in table 1.1 below. Calculate the total white cell percentage of each.

D.   Volu-Sol™ STAT Stain Procedure

1. Obtain three staining dishes or jars. Fill one with STAT Stain and the other two with distilled water. Keep the dish containing the stain tightly covered to prevent evaporation.

2. Dip the slide in STAT stain for 10–15 seconds.

3. Dip the slide in the first dish of water for 10–15 seconds, then "swish" the slide in the second dish of water for 25 seconds. If the water in the dishes develops a surface scum or becomes discolored a dark blue, then change the water.

4. Wipe off the back surface of the slide and allow the smear to air dry.

5. Examine the peripheral blood smears. Identify cell types and perform a differential count: count a total of 100 white blood cells, recording the numbers of each type observed in table 1.1 below. Calculate the total white cell percentage of each.

Table 1.1   **Sketch the appearance of each type of leukocyte you find below, and record the number counted. After counting a total of 100 white cells, calculate the percentage of each.**

NEUTROPHILS	LYMPHOCYTES	MONOCYTES	EOSINOPHILS	BASOPHILS
Totals:				
Percent:				

Table 1.2   Characteristics of Human Peripheral Blood Cells

	Cell Type	Cells/μl Blood	Function	Morphology
	erythrocytes	6×10^6	O_2 transport	concave discs, no nuclei, pink
	platelets	3×10^5	blood clotting and blood vessel repair	small, irregular, red granules with blue cytoplasm
	neutrophils	5,000 (50–70%)	phagocytosis	purple granules, 4-lobe nuclei, size: 9–12 μ
	lymphocytes	3,000 (20–30%)	specific immunity	large round nucleus, blue cytoplasm, size: 7–13 μ
	monocytes	500 (2–6%)	phagocytosis, present antigens	convoluted nucleus, granules, size: 14–18 μ
	eosinophils	300 (1–5%)	destroy antibody-antigen complexes, fight parasites	bright reddish-orange granules, size: 9–12 μ
	basophils	30 (<1%)	may prevent clotting in inflammation	deep purple granules, size: 9–12 μ

Key Terms:

antigen
antibody
primary lymphoid organ
secondary lymphoid organ
lymphatic vessels
hemopoesis
bone marrow
thymus
spleen
lymph node
"MALT"
granulocyte
lymphocyte
"PMN"
leukocyte
eosinophil
neutrophil
monocyte
macrophage
mast cell
basophil
erythrocyte

Questions:

1. What is the most numerous type of leukocyte in human blood? What is this cell's primary function?

2. Were your percentages for human blood within the expected range?

3. Name two areas of the body where lymph nodes can be found. Explain how the location and structure of lymph nodes relate to their function in immunity.

4. Name two characteristics of the spleen.

Additional Reading:

General texts on immunology

1. Silverstein, A. M. 1989. A History of Immunology. New York: Academic Press.

2. Golub, E. 1987. Immunology: A Synthesis. Sunderland, Massachusetts: Sinauer Assoc. Inc.

3. Benjamini and Leskowitz 1991. Immunology: A Short Course. New York: Wiley-Liss.

Journals and Magazines

1. *Immunology Today* (especially good for general reading)

2. *Science*

3. *Scientific American*

4. *Immunological Reviews*

5. *Advances in Immunology*

6. *Journal of Immunology*

7. *Immunology*

Specific Topics:

1. Duijvestijn, A., and A. Hamann. 1989. Mechanisms and regulation of lymphocyte migration. Immunol. Today 10:1–23.

2. Golde, D. W., and J. C. Gasson. 1988. Hormones that stimulate the growth of blood cells. Sci. Am. 259(1):62.

3. Zucker, M. B. 1980. The functioning of blood platelets. Sci. Am. 242(6):70.

4. Rennie, J. 1990. The body against itself. Sci. Am. 263(6):106.

5. Golde, D. W. 1991. The stem cell. Sci. Am. 256(6):86.

6. Tonegawa, S. 1985. The molecules of the immune system. Sci. Am. 253(4):122.

7. Barclay, A. N. 1982. The organization of B and T lymphocytes in lymph nodes. Immunol. Today 3:330–331.

8. Shortman, K. 1984. T cell development in the thymus. Nature 309:583–584.

2 Phagocytosis and Microbial Killing by Macrophages

Phagocytes are cells which ingest and destroy foreign material (such as bacteria), debris and irritants (like asbestos particles) and dead host tissue cells. The process of phagocytosis was first described by the Russian scientist Elie Metchnikoff (the "father of phagocytosis") in the late 1800's. Metchnikoff observed that when the starfish he was studying was pricked with a thorn, cells inside the starfish would rapidly migrate to the site of injury and injest the bacteria found at the wound. We now know that ingestion and killing of bacteria by phagocytes can occur even before the appearance of antibody or other components of specific immunity and is a vitally important front-line defense against infection. Phagocytic defects can result in serious diseases such as Chediak-Higashi syndrome or chronic granulomatous disease. Patients with these illnesses are highly susceptible to infection even by organisms that are usually of very low virulence.

The major phagocytic cell of the bloodstream is the neutrophil, which was seen in exercise 1. The major phagocytic cell of the tissues is the macrophage. Macrophages arise from monocytes in the bloodstream. Monocytes squeeze between cells in the blood vessel walls to enter the tissues and become macrophages. The migration of monocytes out of the blood vessels is called **diapedesis**. Both monocytes and neutrophils diapedese to the tissues to join macrophages already present in the tissues when infections occur.

Macrophages are found widely scattered throughout the connective tissues, where they may survive for weeks or even months. "Resident" macrophages are also found in the tissue of many organs, such as the liver, spleen, lymph nodes, and lungs. Some macrophages ("wandering macrophages") are also capable of migrating to a site of infection. Special phagocytes called microglial cells are found in the central nervous system, where macrophages do not occur.

When an infection occurs in the body tissue, neutrophils and other blood cells migrate to the area via diapedesis, but these cells are quite short-lived. Therefore, the tissue macrophages are very important for removal of foreign particles or dead cell debris. In this exercise, you will induce macrophages to migrate to the abdominal (peritoneal) cavity of a mouse by injecting a sterile irritant into the cavity. You will then harvest the macrophages from the mouse and expose them to bacteria. At several time points you will compare the ability of macrophages to kill bacteria both in the presence of blood serum (the fluid part of blood), and on their own. You will also determine what effect the serum alone has on the bacteria. The bactericidal effects of serum will be explored in greater depth in the next exercise.

Materials:

- ☐ mouse
- ☐ 2 mls "aged" (2 to 3 month old) thioglycollate medium
- ☐ 1-ml syringe and 25 to 27 gauge needle
- ☐ overnight nutrient broth culture of *Staphylococcus* or *Bacillus* species
- ☐ mouse jar with anesthetic and cotton balls
- ☐ dissecting board, scissors, and forceps
- ☐ 70% ethanol in a squirt bottle
- ☐ jar of 95% ethanol
- ☐ 50 mls Hank's Balanced Salt Solution (HBSS)
- ☐ 10 mls cold HBSS
- ☐ 10-ml syringe and 22-gauge needle
- ☐ sterile plugged Pasteur pipette
- ☐ 1 large sterile test tube

- [ ] 36 small sterile test tubes
- [ ] 50 mls sterile saline
- [ ] 50 sterile plugged 1-ml pipettes
- [ ] 32 nutrient agar plates
- [ ] bent glass stir rod for spreading plates
- [ ] 4 microscope slides
- [ ] Wright's Stain or Volu-sol™ Stat stain
- [ ] 0.5 ml normal rabbit serum
- [ ] 37°C water bath
- [ ] 37°C incubator (optional)
- [ ] clinical centrifuge

Procedure:

Step 1 is to be done prior to starting the experiment.

1. Inject the mouse with the 2 mls of thio-glycollate *four days prior to doing this experiment*. The mouse should be injected intraperitoneally (see fig. 2.1). Your instructor will assist you with the injection. Also inoculate a broth culture with bacteria the day before the experiment.

2. On the day of the experiment, prepare the bacterial culture by centrifuging at $1800 \times g$ for 20 minutes. Discard the supernatant from the bacterial pellet and wash the bacteria in a volume of HBSS equal to the original culture volume. Centrifuge the bacteria again and resus-

pend in HBSS. Using McFarland standards (Appendix 3, #16, p. 194), dilute enough of the culture in HBSS to make 2 to 5 mls at a concentration of 1×10^7 cells/ml.

3. To begin the experiment, euthanize the mouse by placing it in a jar or coffee can with a couple of anesthetic-soaked cotton balls. Close the jar tightly and wait 5 minutes.

4. After the mouse has died, place it on a dissecting board and wet down the fur with 70% ethanol. Cut open just the outer skin and muscle layers of the abdomen, using ethanol-flamed scissors and forceps. Be very careful not to cut through the peritoneal membrane around the abdominal cavity, which lies just under the abdominal skin and muscle. Keep the tip of the scissors pointed upwards while cutting through the skin to avoid cutting the underlying membrane.

5. Inject 10 mls of cold HBSS through the peritoneal membrane and into the abdominal cavity. The peritoneal membrane will stretch somewhat as you fill up the cavity. Holding the mouse down firmly at the chest, begin gently shaking

---

⚠ **Safety Tips:**
1. **Avoid breathing anesthetic vapors.**
2. **Use caution when handling syringes. Remember to never re-cap a syringe or lay it on the bench. Place the syringe in an empty tube if you must put it down.**
3. **Some *Staphylococcus* species are potential pathogens. Avoid aerosolization from syringes. Always cover the tip of the needle with an alcohol-soaked cotton ball when expressing fluid from the syringe.**
4. **Be careful not to let ethanol drip down onto your hand when flaming dissection tools, and do not place hot dissection tools directly into the ethanol or touch the ethanol-doused mouse.**
5. **If an ethanol fire does occur, don't panic or use water, but simply smother the fire with a beaker or towel.**
6. **Wright's stain is a flammable poison. Keep it away from sparks or flames. The vapor is harmful if inhaled.**

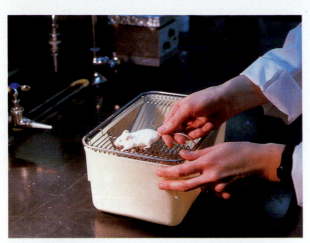

A. Hold the mouse at the base of the tail with your right hand (if you are right-handed) and let it pull away from you on the top of its cage.

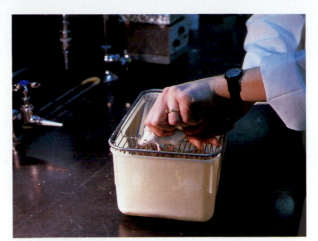

B. Using your thumb and the knuckle of your first finger, pinch tightly together the loose skin around the neck just over the ears.

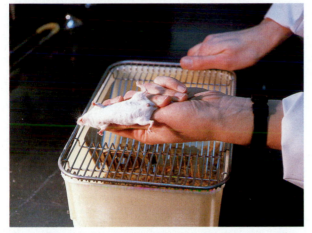

C. Stretch the mouse out taughtly in your palm and pin its tail under your ring finger.

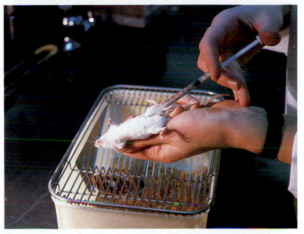

D. With the mouse's head held downwards, inject the mouse in the left lower abdomen.

Figure 2.1   Intraperitoneal Injection of the Mouse.

and massaging the lower half of the mouse carcass to help loosen peritoneal macrophages from the walls of the abdomen. Continue shaking the mouse for about 3 minutes.

6. Have a sterile Pasteur pipette and bulb ready to use (set in a sterile tube in a rack). Pull up on the peritoneal membrane using an ethanol-flamed forceps while making a small snip through the membrane with a scissors held in your other hand. Do not release your forceps grip on the membrane as you insert the

Pasteur pipette through the snip in the membrane and aspirate fluid from the abdominal cavity. Transfer this fluid to a sterile test tube. The fluid should appear somewhat turbid due to the cells suspended in it.

7. Label 4 test tubes "A," "B," "C," and "D." Prepare the following mixtures in the tubes and incubate all tubes for 1 hour in a 37°C water bath. Note that tube A is the test for phagocytosis, and tubes B, C, and D are experimental controls.

Tube	A	B	C	D
serum	0.2 ml	0.2 ml	—	—
cells	1 ml	—	1 ml	—
bacteria	0.5 ml	0.5 ml	0.5 ml	0.5 ml
HBSS	0.3 ml	1.3 ml	0.5 ml	1.5 ml

8. During the 1 hour incubation, prepare eight dilution blanks, each containing 0.9 mls saline, for each test tube A–D. Also label eight nutrient agar plates for each tube A–D. You should have 32 dilution blanks and 32 plates total. See figure 2.2 for a diagram of this procedure.

9. After the 1 hour incubation period, spread a drop from each tube A–D on each of four microscope slides to make smears. Allow the slides to air dry.

10. Make ten-fold serial dilutions of each of the tubes A–D through eight saline dilution blanks. To do this, transfer 0.1 ml from tube A into the first of the eight dilution blanks. This is a 1:10, or 10^{-1}, dilution. Mix the first blank, then transfer 0.1 ml from it to the second dilution blank. This is a 1:100, or 10^{-2} dilution. Mix the second blank and transfer 0.1 ml from it to the third dilution blank, and so on. Continue making ten-fold dilutions through the eighth tube. Repeat this dilution scheme with tubes B–D.

11. Transfer 0.1 ml from the first dilution blank for tube A to a nutrient agar plate labeled "A—dilution 1:10." Spread the inoculum on the plate using a bent glass rod that has been dipped in 95% ethanol and passed through the bunsen burner flame. Be sure to allow the rod to cool before placing it in the inoculum. It is not necessary to "bake" the rod in the flame. Simply passing it through to ignite the ethanol is sufficient to sterilize

the rod. Also make sure that you keep spreading the inoculum until it has been completely absorbed by the agar.

12. Continue spreading 0.1 ml from each dilution blank onto the appropriate plate, flaming the glass rod between each plate.

13. Stain the microscope slides with Wright's stain as described in exercise 1. Look for phagocytized bacteria within the cells. The bacteria will stain a dark purple with the wright's stain.

14. Invert the plates and incubate them at 37°C for 24 to 48 hours. Following incubation, count the number of colonies on "countable" plates (preferrably those having between 30 and 100 colonies). Calculate colony forming units per ml, or "CFU/ml" for each of the tubes A–D. Record your results below.

RESULTS

Tube	Viable bacteria (# bacteria surviving per ml)
A	
B	
C	
D	

Key Terms:
phagocytosis
diapedesis
monocyte
macrophage
microglial cell
peritoneal cavity

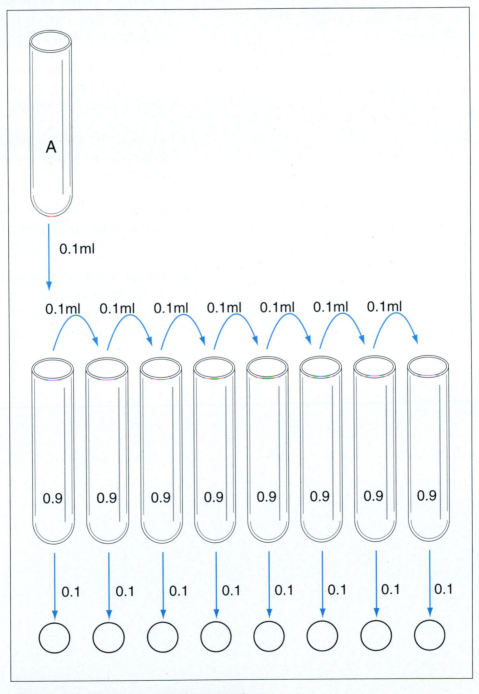

Figure 2.2   Diagram of dilution procedure

Questions:

1. What are three differences between macrophages and neutrophils?

2. Where are some locations in the body where fixed tissue macrophages can be found?

3. What is the function of phagocytes in innate immunity?

Additional Reading:

1. Van Furth, R. 1985. Mononuclear phagocytes—Characteristics, Physiology and Function. Boston: Martinus Nijhoff.

2. Cline, M. J., R. I. Lehrer, M. C. Territo, and D. W. Golde. 1978. Monocytes and macrophages: functions and diseases. Ann. Intern. Med. 88:78–88.

3. Babior, B. M. 1978. Oxygen-dependent microbial killing by phagocytes. N. Engl. J. Med. 298:659–668, 721–725.

4. Elsbach, P. 1980. Degradation of micro-organisms by phagocytic cells. Rev. Inf. Dis. 2:106.

5. Gabig, T. G., and B. M. Babior. 1981. The killing of pathogens by phagocytes. Ann. Rev. Med. 32:313–326.

6. Stossel, T. P., R. K. Root, and M. Vaughan. 1972. Phagocytosis in chronic granulomatous disease and the Chediak-Higashi syndrome. N. Engl. J. Med. 286:120–123.

3 Bactericidal Effects of Normal Serum

Plasma is the fluid portion of the blood in which all the blood cells are suspended. If both the cells and the clotting factors are removed by allowing the blood to clot, the yellowish fluid that remains is call **serum**. Serum is a mixture of many different soluble factors and proteins. Serum from individuals who have been vaccinated or exposed to infectious agents contains specific disease-fighting proteins called antibodies, which will be considered later. In this exercise you will observe the effects of some of the innate components of serum that are capable of fighting infections even if an individual has not yet been vaccinated or previously exposed.

The innate bactericidal effects of serum were first observed by Pfeiffer in 1894. Pfeiffer discovered that cholera bacilli were "dissolved" when mixed with normal serum. He also found that this lytic activity of serum could be destroyed by simply heating the serum at 56°C for 30 minutes. We now know that fresh serum contains a group of proteins called "complement." These heat-labile proteins are capable of lysing gram negative bacteria and, once activated, also generate other bioactive substances that cause dilation of blood vessels, increased capillary flow, and chemotaxis of phagocytes. You can probably see how the complement proteins can aid the phagocytic response to infecting microbes.

Serum contains many other naturally occurring factors besides complement that are involved in immunity. These include properdin, C-reactive protein, fibrinogen, and interferon (an antiviral substance) to name a few. The combined effect of the soluble serum components, both innate and specific, is known as **humoral** immunity.

Materials:

- [ ] overnight broth culture of a gram positive bacterial species
- [ ] overnight broth culture of a gram negative bacterial species
- [ ] 1 ml normal rabbit serum
- [ ] 55 sterile test tubes
- [ ] 60 mls sterile saline
- [ ] 48 nutrient agar plates
- [ ] 60 sterile, cotton-plugged 1-ml pipettes
- [ ] bent glass rod for spreading plates
- [ ] jar containing 95% ethanol
- [ ] 37°C water bath
- [ ] 56°C water bath
- [ ] 37°C incubator (optional)

Procedure:

Broth cultures are to be prepared the day prior to starting the experiment.

1. Place 1 ml of the serum sample provided in a sterile test tube and incubate it at 56°C for 30 minutes. Reserve the remaining 1 ml of serum at room temperature.

2. Label six tubes A–F. Starting with the gram positive culture, mix 0.5 mls of the culture with 0.5 mls of heated serum in tube A. Mix 0.5 mls of the culture with 0.5 mls of unheated, normal serum in tube B. Mix 0.5 mls of the culture with 0.5 mls of saline in tube C. Repeat with the gram negative culture for tubes D, E, and F. You should have six tubes total. Note that tubes C and F are negative controls.

3. Incubate all six tubes in a 37°C water bath for 1 hour. Meanwhile, prepare eight dilution blanks, each containing

0.9 mls saline, for each of the six tubes. You will have a total of 48 dilution blanks. Also label eight plates with the dilutions (10^{-1} through 10^{-8}) for each of the six incubating tubes. See figure 3.1 for a diagram of the dilution procedure.

4. After incubation, prepare serial ten-fold dilutions of each of the six tubes as follows. Transfer 0.1 ml from incubation tube A into the first of the eight dilution blanks. This is a 1:10, or 10-1, dilution. Mix the first blank, then transfer 0.1 ml from it to the second dilution blank. This is a 1:100, or 10-2 dilution. Mix the second blank and transfer 0.1 ml from it to the third dilution blank, and so on. Continue making ten-fold dilutions through the eighth tube. Repeat for tubes B–F.

5. Transfer 0.1 ml from the first dilution blank to the appropriately labeled nutrient agar plate. Spread the inoculum on the plate using a bent glass rod that has been dipped in 95% ethanol and passed through the bunsen burner flame. Be sure to allow the rod to cool before placing it in the inoculum. It is not necessary to "bake" the rod in the flame. Simply passing it through to ignite the ethanol is sufficient to sterilize the rod. Also make sure that you keep spreading the inoculum until it has been completely absorbed by the agar.

6. Continue spreading 0.1 ml from each dilution blank onto the appropriate plate, flaming the glass rod between each plate.

7. Invert the plates and incubate them at 37°C for 24 to 48 hours. Following incubation, count the number of colonies on "countable" plates (preferrably those having between 30 and 100 colonies). Calculate colony forming units per ml, or "CFU/ml" for each of the six tubes. Record your results below.

Tube	Viable bacteria (# bacteria surviving per ml)
A	
B	
C	
D	
E	
F	

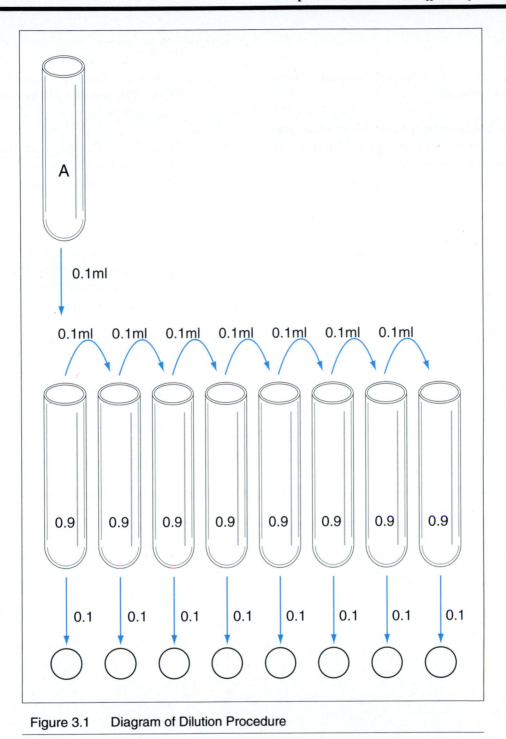

Figure 3.1   Diagram of Dilution Procedure

Key Terms:
  complement
  humoral immuity

Questions:

1. What is the difference between plasma and serum?

2. What is complement? Give three reasons why complement is important to the immune system.

3. What are some other soluble immune factors besides complement that are present in normal serum?

Additional Reading:

1. Muller-Eberhard, H. J., and H. R. Colton. 1986. The complement system. Prog. Immunol. 6:267.

2. Fearon, D. T., and K. F. Austen. 1980. The alternative pathway of complement—a system for host resistance to microbial infection. N. Engl. J. Med. 303:259.

3. Muschel, L. H., and H. P. Treffers. 1953. Quantitative studies on the bactericidal actions of serum and complement. J. Immunol. 76:1–10.

4. Bloom, B. R. 1980. Interferons and the immune system. Nature 284:593–595.

5. Ninnemann, J. L. 1984. Prostaglandins and immunity. Immunol. Today 5:170–178.

6. Kushner, I., H. Gewurz, and M. D. Benson. 1981. C-reactive protein and the acute-phase response. J. Lab. Clin. Med. 97:739–749.

4 Nonspecific Immunity -- Clearance of Infection by Mice

Protection against disease involves several specific immune activities such as antibody formation by B-cell lymphocytes, and cellular activities mediated by T-cell lymphocytes and other cells. A specific immune response is one which involves a recognition of a specific antigen, response to that antigen, and memory of the antigen should it be encountered again. However, there are also **nonspecific**, or **natural** immune activities which usually act as a first line defense. It is only when microorganisms are able to evade these initial defenses that the specific immune functions are called into play.

Nonspecific immunity is a combination of barriers which hinder the invasion of microorganisms; including physical or mechanical barriers such as the skin, mucous secretions and cilia lining the respiratory tract, the cough and sneeze reflexes, low pH of the skin, stomach, and vaginal tract, and competition from normal flora; cellular barriers such as the phagocytes; as well as molecular barriers such as lysozyme in the tears, serum complement proteins and interferons.

The phagocytic cells consist of both **wandering** and **fixed** cells. Both types are responsible for engulfing and digesting foreign particles in the body. The body's entire complement of phagocytic cells and the organs in which they reside are sometimes referred to as the **reticuloendothelial system**. Wandering phagocytes include both the polymorphonuclear leukocytes (neutrophils or "PMNs") of the blood and the tissue macrophages studied in exercise 2. These are "standby" cells which can be called by chemical signals to a localized site of infection. The fixed phagocytes are usually found in blood-filtering organs such as the liver, spleen, and lungs, and have been given different names depending on the organ in which they reside. For example, the resident phagocytes of the liver are sometimes called "Kupffer cells," and the phagocytes of the lungs are called "dust cells." These cells are very efficient at clearing invading microbes from the blood or lymph, and can do so very quickly. Any time there is a break in the skin barrier which allows infecting organisms to enter, such as a prick in the finger, **inflammation** results. The characteristic redness, swelling, heat, and pain (known as the four cardinal signs of inflammation), result in part from the accumulation of fluid and phagocytic cells which have been called to the site of infection. The PMNs are usually the first to arrive, but are short-lived. Macrophages are slower but longer-lived. Pus is actually an accumulation of PMNs which have died.

Not all invading microorganisms are phagocytized at the same rate. Some bacteria have surface features, such as a capsule, which allows them to resist phagocytosis. Infections by these organisms may be more difficult to resolve unless specific antibody is formed. Once antibody has been produced, it coats the microbe and renders it more susceptible to phagocytosis. This process is called **opsonization**.

In this exercise, mice will be exposed to infecting bacteria. The rate of clearance of the bacteria from the bloodstream and the location of the bacteria after clearance will be explored. The mice will be injected intravenously with a bacterial suspension, then euthanized at timed intervals. Samples of peripheral blood, and tissue from the spleen and liver are diluted and plated to determine bacterial numbers.

⚠ *Safety Tips:*
1. **Avoid breathing anesthetic vapors.**
2. **Use caution when handling syringes. Never re-cap a syringe or lay it on the bench. Place the syringe in an empty tube if you must put it down.**
3. ***Serratia* is a potential pathogen. Avoid aerosolization from syringes. Always cover the tip of the needle with an alcohol-soaked cotton ball when expressing fluid from the syringe.**
4. **Be careful not to let ethanol drip down onto your hand when flaming dissection tools, and do not place hot dissection tools directly into the ethanol or touch the ethanol-doused mouse.**
5. **If an ethanol fire does occur, don't panic or use water, but simply smother the fire with a beaker or towel.**

Materials:

- ☐ 6 mice
- ☐ overnight nutrient broth culture of *Serratia marcescens*
- ☐ 50 mls sterile saline in a bottle
- ☐ 1 sterile test tube or stoppered vial
- ☐ mouse restraining device and heat lamp
- ☐ small bottle of 70% ethanol and cotton balls
- ☐ 1 ml syringes with 27-gauge needles
- ☐ food coloring dyes for marking mice
- ☐ mouse jar with anesthetic and cotton balls
- ☐ dissecting board, scissors, and forceps
- ☐ 70% ethanol in a squirt bottle
- ☐ jar of 95% ethanol
- ☐ sterile plugged Pasteur pipette
- ☐ 4 sterile beakers or petri plates
- ☐ 2 sterile mortar and pestles
- ☐ 36 0.9 ml sterile saline dilution blanks
- ☐ 36 nutrient agar plates
- ☐ 40 1.0 ml sterile plugged pipettes
- ☐ bent glass rod for spreading plates
- ☐ weighing scale
- ☐ 37°C shaking water bath

Procedure:

Step 1 must be performed the day prior to the exercise.

1. The day before the exercise, inoculate a flask of nutrient broth from a culture of *Serratia marcescens*, and incubate overnight in a shaking water bath at 37°C.

2. Dilute the broth culture by adding 0.1 ml culture to 9.9 mls sterile saline (a 1:100 dilution) in a tube or vial. Use this suspension for injecting the mice. Also label six 0.9 ml saline dilution blanks and six nutrient agar plates for each time point for blood, liver, and spleen. (Note—each lab group is responsible for one of the time points). See figure 4.1 for a diagram of the experimental prcoedure.

3. You will follow the scheme for injection and timing outlined in table 4.1. Each mouse will represent a different timed interval. The "0 time" mouse will receive an injection of plain saline with no bacteria. This will mean keeping each mouse in a separate cage or marking each with food color so you can keep track of them. You will record the injection time for each mouse as each injection is completed.

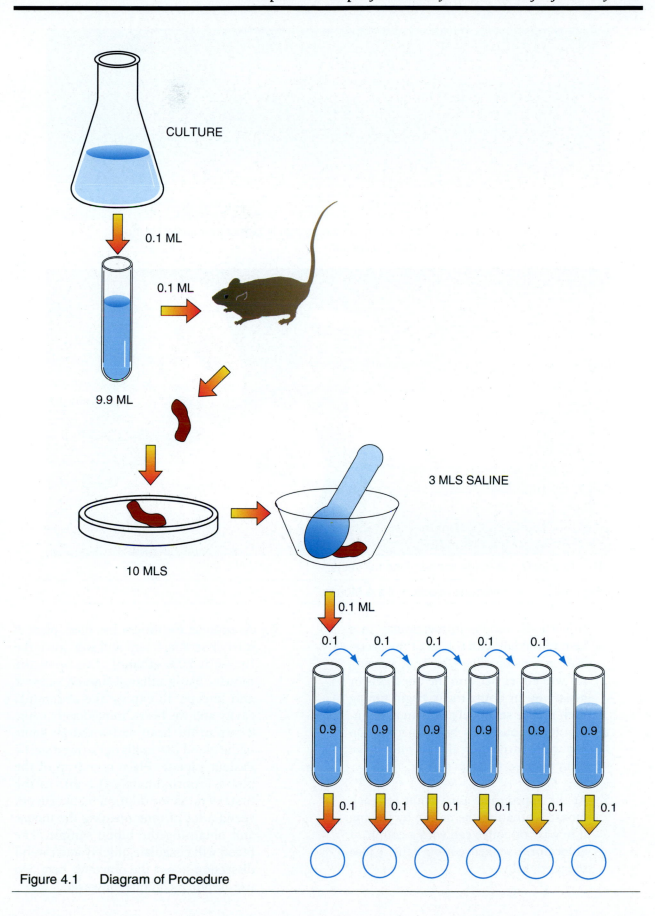

Figure 4.1   Diagram of Procedure

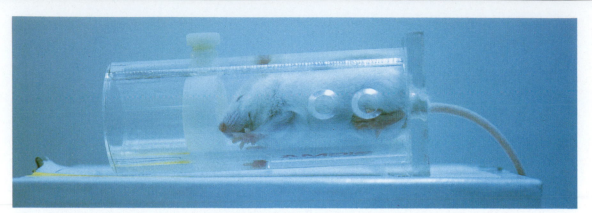

A. The mouse is placed in a restraining device so that it cannot be injured by the experimentor by struggling during injection.

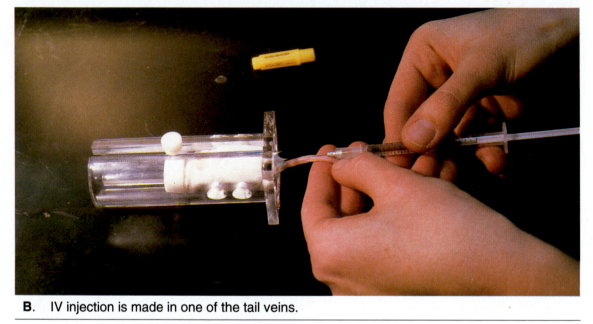

B. IV injection is made in one of the tail veins.

Figure 4.2   Intravenous Injection of the Mouse.

4. Inject each mouse intravenously in a vein of the tail with 0.1 ml of the bacterial suspension (fig. 4.2). Your instructor will either perform the injections or assist you in doing them. Begin timing each mouse separately as soon as an individual mouse has been injected. Do *not* wait until after all the mice have been injected to begin timing.

5. At the appropriate time point for each mouse, euthanize the mouse by placing it in a jar or coffee can with a couple of chloroform-soaked cotton balls. Close the jar tightly.

6. As soon as the mouse has died, place it on a dissecting board and wet down the fur with 70% ethanol. Cut open the mouse, using ethanol-flamed scissors and forceps, to expose the abdominal cavity and the heart. Immediately make a snip in the heart and withdraw some of the blood that spills out using a sterile Pasteur pipette. Place one drop of the blood (approximately 0.1 ml) in the first 0.9 ml saline dilution blank. Do not spend a lot of time opening the mouse and obtaining the blood sample. The blood will coagulate quickly and careful dissection is not the objective here. Do use aseptic technique, however.

7. Remove the liver and the spleen and place each in separate sterile beakers or petri plates. Add 10 mls of sterile saline to each to wash any peripheral blood off the organs.

8. Transfer each organ to a second sterile container. Cut off a piece of each organ equal to 0.1 to 0.5 grams. Record the weight of each piece and place in separate mortar and pestles.

9. Add 5 mls saline to each mortar. Grind each organ to a smooth suspension to release the bacteria trapped in the organ.

10. Transfer 0.1 mls from the spleen suspension to the first 0.9 ml saline dilution blank with a 1-ml pipette. Mix the tube and with a new 1-ml pipette, transfer 0.1 mls from the first dilution blank to the second dilution blank.

11. Using a new pipette for each transfer, serially dilute through the remaining four spleen dilution blanks by transferring 0.1 ml. You should now have six tenfold dilutions of spleen suspension. Repeat steps 10 and 11 for the six dilutions of liver suspension and the remaining five dilutions of blood.

12. Place 0.1 ml of each dilution for each organ and the blood on separate labeled nutrient agar plates. You may use the same pipette if you work from the most dilute tube back to the most concentrated tube, but you must change pipettes between each organ and the blood. Spread the drops on the plates with an ethanol flamed bent glass rod, again working backwards from the most dilute sample. Make sure that you continue spreading until all the liquid has been absorbed by the agar.

13. Repeat steps 5–12 for each time point. Incubate all the plates at room temperature for two days. Count the number of colonies on plates which show between 30 and 300 colonies. *Serratia* colonies will exhibit a red pigment when incubated at room temperature. Calculate the number of bacteria per ml blood and the number of bacteria per gram liver and spleen for each time point. Plot your values on a semi-log graph.

Table 4.1   Experiment 4 schedule

mouse #	time point (min.) after injection	dilutions of blood or organ suspension to plate
1 (no bact.)	0	10^{-1} to 10^{-6}
2	10	
3	20	
4	30	
5	40	
6	60	

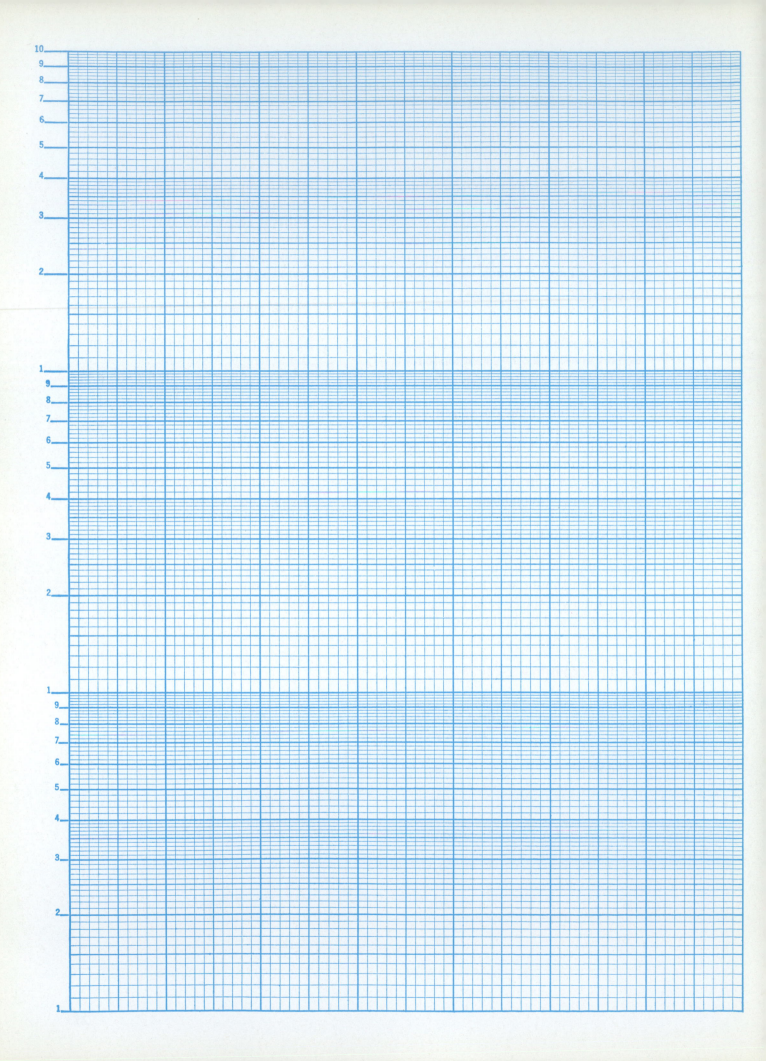

Key Terms:

natural immunity
nonspecific immunity
fixed and wandering phagocytes
reticuloendothelial system
Kupffer cells and dust cells
inflammation
opsonization

Questions:

1. What is the function of the reticuloendothelial system?

2. Describe the route that microorganisms would take as they escape phagocytosis in the tissues and eventually end up causing a bacteremia?

2. What is opsonization and how does this process help the immune system resist infection by some organisms?

3. Design an experiment to test the difference in clearance rates between an encapsulated bacteria, like *Klebsiella pneumonia* and an organism which lacks a capsule, like *Serratia marcescens*.

4. How would you design an experiment to test whether the presence of antibodies against *Klebsiella* increases the rate of clearance?

5. Why must you change pipettes between tubes when making dilutions? Why is it permissible to use the same pipette when transferring 0.1 mls from each dilution tube to the plates?

Additional Reading:

1. Larsen, G. L. and P. M. Henson. 1983. Mediators of inflammation. Ann. Rev. Immunol. 1:335.

2. Edelson, R. L., and J. M. Fink. 1985. The immunologic function of skin. Sci. Am. 252(6):46.

3. Hay, J. B., and B. B. Hobb. 1977. The flow of blood to lymph nodes and its relation to lymphocyte traffic and the immune response. J. Exp. Med. 145:31–44.

5 Separation of Peripheral Blood Components

Peripheral blood is the usual source of lymphoid cells for studies of the human immune system. A simple and rapid method for purifying the mononuclear cell fraction (containing lymphocytes and monocytes) of peripheral blood involves centrifugation of the blood through a Ficoll-Hypaque density gradient (fig. 5.1). This method takes advantage of the density differences between different cellular components of the blood. Mononuclear cells, which have a low density, collect in the first band near the top of the gradient, while the more dense granulocytes and erythrocytes pellet at the bottom of the tube. Monocytes can be separated from the lymphocytes by placing the cells in a tissue culture flask. Monocytes will adhere to the flask while the lymphocytes will remain in suspension.

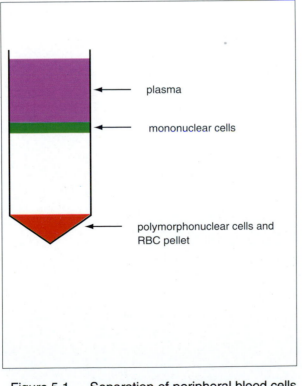

Figure 5.1   Separation of peripheral blood cells on a Ficoll-Hypaque gradient

plasma

mononuclear cells

polymorphonuclear cells and RBC pellet

Materials:

- [ ] 5 mls of heparinized peripheral blood
- [ ] 4 15-ml centrifuge tubes
- [ ] 5 mls Phosphate-buffered saline (PBS)
- [ ] 3 mls of Ficoll-Hypaque solution
- [ ] 3 microscope slides and coverslips
- [ ] Wright's stain and Wright's buffer
- [ ] 2 Pasteur pipettes
- [ ] 4 10-ml pipettes
- [ ] clinical centrifuge

Procedure:

1. Collect 5 mls of peripheral blood in a tube containing 1 unit of sodium-heparin. The blood may be obtained from a rabbit as outlined in exercise 9, or human blood can be used if the mononuclear cells isolated in this exercise will be used for exercise 6.

2. Transfer the heparinized blood to a centrifuge tube and add an equal volume of PBS. Mix well.

3. Add 3 mls of Ficoll-Hypaque mixture to a second centrifuge tube. Slowly layer the 10 mls of blood/PBS mixture on top of the Ficoll-Hypaque, being careful to maintain the interface between the two layers.

4. Centrifuge 30 minutes at 900 × g at room temp. with no brake.

5. With a 10-ml pipette, carefully remove the upper layer containing the plasma and most of the platelets. Place a drop of this layer on a microscope slide. Spread the drop around to make a smear and allow to air dry.

⚠ *Safety Tips:*

1. **If human blood is used for this experiment, gloves and safety goggles must be worn.**
2. **Wright's stain is a flammable poison. Keep it away from sparks or flames. The vapor is harmful if inhaled.**

6. Using a Pasteur pipette, transfer the mononuclear cell layer to another centrifuge tube. Save this fraction if it is to be used for isolating T cells in exercise 6. Also make a smear from one drop of this cell layer on a microscope slide for later staining.

7. Make a smear from the polymorphonuclear cell layer of the centrifuge tube.

8. Stain the smears prepared in steps 5–7 with Wright's stain (as in ex. 1), and observe the cell types present.

Key Terms:

density gradient
Ficoll-Hypaque
heparin

Additional Reading:

1. Mishell, B. B. and S. M. Shiigi, eds. 1980. Selected Methods in Cellular Immunology. San Francisco: W. H. Freeman and Co.

2. Coligan, J. E., et al., eds. 1991. Current Protocols in Immunology. New York: Greene Publishing Associates and Wiley-Interscience.

3. Boyum, A. 1968. Isolation of mononuclear cells and granulocytes from human blood. Scand. J. Clin. Lab. Invest. Suppl. 21:77–89.

6   T-cell Rosettes

There are many procedures available for isolating specific cell populations from the blood or lymphoid organs. These procedures may be required for certain studies, such as the study of the distribution of specific surface markers on cells, the function of specific groups of B-cells or T-cells, or deficiencies in the immune response due to defects in particular cell types. Both depletion of cell populations and positive selection of cell populations can be used to fractionate a mixture of cell types.

Erythrocytes can be removed from a cell population by hypotonic lysis. Adherent cells like monocytes can be removed by adherence to the surface of a flask, or by passing the cell mixture over a nylon wool column. Both monocytes and B-cells will adhere to the nylon wool. B-cells have surface-bound antibody (immunoglobulin, or "Ig"), and may be removed from a mixture by placing the cell mixture in a petri plate which has been coated with anti-Ig antibody. The B-cells will be bound by the anti-Ig via their surface immunoglobulin molecules. This method is called B-cell **panning**. T-cells can also be removed by panning techniques using petri plates coated with antibody directed against specific T-cell surface antigens. Monocytes, B-cells, and T-cells can all be removed from a cell mixture by elimination with cytotoxic antibodies. This method is explored in exercise 25. All these methods operate by negative selection, because the relevant cell types are depleted from the mixture.

In the following exercise you will use a positive selection technique for isolating T-cells. T-cells will spontaneously bind to and form **rosettes** with sheep red blood cells. The rosettes can be seen under the microscope, and can be separated from unbound B-cells and monocytes by Ficoll-Hypaque centrifugation.

Materials:

- [ ] mononuclear cell fraction of human peripheral blood
- [ ] 50 mls Hank's Balanced Salt Solution (HBSS)
- [ ] 0.5 mls calf serum (heat-inactivated at 56°C for 30 min. to remove complement, and absorbed with sheep RBCs)
- [ ] 1 ml sheep blood in Alsever's solution (20% red blood cells)
- [ ] 70% ethanol
- [ ] hemocytometer
- [ ] 2 test tubes
- [ ] 4 15-ml centrifuge tubes
- [ ] Pasteur pipettes
- [ ] 1-ml pipettes
- [ ] 10-ml pipettes
- [ ] ice bucket
- [ ] 37°C water bath
- [ ] 56°C water bath

⚠ **Safety Tip:**
Because human blood is used for this experiment, gloves and safety goggles must be worn.

Part A: T-cell Rosettes

Procedure:

1. Obtain the mononuclear cell fraction from peripheral blood, and place in a 15-ml centrifuge tube. The cells may be obtained by the procedure outlined in exercise 5. Add HBSS to the mononuclear cells to a volume of 15 mls. At the same time, add 1 ml of sheep blood to a 15-ml centrifuge and fill to the 15 mls with HBSS. Centrifuge both tubes for 10

minutes at 1000 × g. Remove the supernatant from the monocytes by decanting off the liquid. Remove the supernatant from the sheep erythrocytes using a pipette, because these cells will not form a hard pellet.

2. Resuspend the mononuclear cells again in 15 mls of HBSS. Set aside 0.5 mls of this cell suspension and count these cells in a hemocytometer using trypan blue staining (see part B). Resuspend the sheep blood pellet to 15 mls in HBSS. Centrifuge both tubes again as before. While the cells are spinning, use your hemocytometer counts to calculate the volume of HBSS you will need to resuspend the mononuclear cells to a concentration of 1×10^6 cells per ml.

3. Prepare a 0.5 ml suspension of mononuclear cells in HBSS at a concentration of about 1×10^6 cells/ml in a centrifuge tube as calculated. Resuspend the sheep blood pellet to prepare 0.5 mls of a 0.5% concentration in HBSS.

4. Add 0.5 ml of calf serum and 0.5 ml of 0.5% sheep blood to the 0.5 mls mononuclear cells.

5. Incubate the mixture 10 minutes in a 37°C water bath, then centrifuge 5 minutes at 200 × g. Do not remove the supernatant or disturb the cell pellet. Incubate the tube at least 1 hour or up to two or three days on ice or in a refrigerator, leaving the supernatant in the tube.

6. *Gently* resuspend the cells by tipping the tube and rotating in a horizontal position for 1 or 2 minutes. Any rough treatment at this point could disrupt the rosettes. Carefully fill the chamber of a hemocytometer with the rosette suspension and observe under the microscope. Rosettes are cells which have bound three or more RBCs.

Part B: Use of the Hemocytometer

1. Mix a small amount of the cell suspension with an equal volume of trypan blue solution. Mix thoroughly by pipetting up and down with a Pasteur pipette, and allow to stand for 10 minutes.

2. Meanwhile, clean the hemocytometer and coverslip with 70% ethanol and lens paper.

3. With the coverslip in place on the hemocytometer, use a Pasteur pipette to transfer the cell suspension/dye mixture to both chambers. Carefully touch the edge of the chamber to the pipette tip and allow the chamber to fill by capillary action. Do not overfill or underfill the chambers.

4. Starting with one chamber, count all the cells in the four 1 mm corner squares (figure 6.1). Keep a separate count of the number of viable cells and dead cells (dead cells stain blue). For cells lying on a line, count those which lie on top or left lines of the squares, but not those which lie on bottom or right lines of the squares.

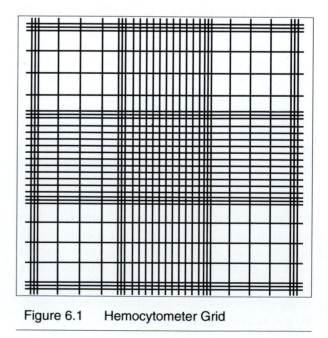

Figure 6.1   Hemocytometer Grid

5. Count the second chamber in the same manner as the first.

6. The hemocytometer chamber represents a volume of 0.1 mm^3, or 1×10^{-4} cm^3. Because 1 cm^3 is equivalent to 1 ml, the cell concentration per ml can be calculated using a chamber volume conversion factor of 10^4 in the equation below:

7. If the cells appear clustered or there is more than 10% variation in the cell counts between chambers, repeat the count after dispersing the cells in the original suspension and then the dye dilution by vigorous pipetting.

8. If there are less than 100 or greater than 400 cells to count (25–100 cells per 1 mm square), repeat the procedure after adjusting the cells to an appropriate dilution (this dilution factor must be taken into account in the calculations).

9. There should not be less than 95% viability of the cells for most procedures.

 # cells/ml = average count per square × dilution factor × chamber conversion factor

e.g., if 200 cells were counted in one chamber from a 1:2 dilution of cells in trypan blue, the number of cells per ml in the original suspension is calculated as:

$$\frac{200\ \textit{cells counted}}{4\ \textit{squares}} \times 2 \times 10^4 = 1 \times 10^6\ \textit{cells/ml}$$

The total number of cells in the original sample is then:

$$\textit{\# cells/ml} \times \textit{total volume of sample (ml)}$$

Which, for a 10 ml suspension would be:

$$1 \times 10^6\ \textit{cells/ml} \times 10\ \textit{ml} = 1 \times 10^7\ \textit{total cells}$$

Key Terms:

immunoglobulin
"panning"
T-cell rosettes

Questions:

1. How might you isolate B-cells from the mononuclear cell population rather than T-cells?

2. What is the receptor on the surface of human T-cells that binds sheep erythrocytes?

Additional Reading:

1. Mishell, B. B. and S. M. Shiigi, eds. 1980. Selected Methods in Cellular Immunology. San Francisco: W. H. Freeman and Co.

2. Coligan, J. E., et al., eds. 1991. Current Protocols in Immunology. New York: Greene Publishing Associates and Wiley-Interscience.

3. Rose, N. R., H. Friedman, and J. L. Fahey, eds. 1986. Manual of Clinical Laboratory Immunology. 3rd ed. American Society for Microbiology.

4. Howard, F. D., et al. 1981. A human T lymphocyte differentiation marker defined by monoclonal antibodies that block E-rosette formation. J. Immunol. 126:2117–2122.

7 Preparation of Tissue-derived Protein Antigens

An antigen must be at least 750 Daltons M. W. and preferably over 10,000 Da to be immunogenic (to elicit an immune response). Most particulate antigens or large complex macromolecules of protein and carbohydrate are good immunogens while nucleic acids and lipids are usually poor immunogens. Although most soluble proteins are immunogenic, when injected directly into the bloodstream they may be cleared from the circulation too quickly for development of a good immune response. Therefore, most protein antigens are first mixed with an insoluble compound called an "adjuvant." This mixture is then injected under the skin or into the muscle, where it is cleared only very slowly from the body and has sufficient time to elicit an immune response. The use of adjuvants will be explored in exercise 9. Very small molecules (haptens) as well as nucleic acids and lipids may be made immunogenic by conjugating them to large carrier proteins (fig. 7.1). In general, the more distant the relationship between the donor of the antigen and the immunized animal, the greater the immune response.

In this exercise you will prepare a protein antigen solution from a tissue source. The antigen solution obtained will actually be a mixture of several tissue proteins.

A. Extraction of Tissue Protein
To extract proteins from the tissue, it is necessary to break down the tissue fibers and allow the proteins to diffuse out of the tissue fragments.

Materials for Part A:
- [ ] tissue source (beef, pork, or chicken from the supermarket)
- [ ] weighing scale
- [ ] scalpel or knife and cutting board
- [ ] mortar and pestle
- [ ] 30 mls saline solution
- [ ] 2 50-ml plastic centrifuge tubes
- [ ] 2 10-ml pipettes
- [ ] stir rod
- [ ] clinical centrifuge

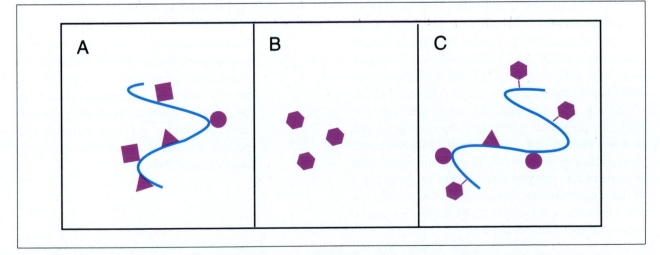

Figure 7.1   Schematic representation of a protein antigen with various antigenic determinants (**A**), a hapten (**B**), and a hapten bound to a carrier protein (**C**).

Procedure:

1. Use a scalpel or knife to cut off a piece of tissue weighing about 10 grams. Cut the tissue into small pieces and place the pieces in a clean mortar and pestle with 10 mls of saline.

2. Grind the tissue until completely pulverized. If the tissue mixture is too thick (like paste), add 10 to 20 more mls of saline until you have a soup-like mixture. Let this mixture sit, with occasional stirring, for 20 to 30 minutes.

3. Decant the tissue mixture into a 50-ml centrifuge tube, and spin at $1800 \times g$ for 15 minutes.

4. After centrifuging, transfer the supernatant (containing protein) to a second centrifuge tube and discard the tissue debris.

B. Equilibrium Dialysis of the Extracted Proteins

After preparing the tissue protein extract, it will be necessary to separate the large protein molecules from small, non-immunogenic molecules by dialysis through membrane tubing. Dialysis tubing is a semipermeable cellulose membrane which allows the separation of molecules by diffusion. The tubing is manufactured in various pore-size ranges. It is easy to separate the large proteins from small molecules by using tubing of pore-size 12,000 to 14,000 molecular weight. When the dialysis tubing is filled with the extract and placed into a buffer solution, the small molecules will pass through the pores and into the buffer by diffusion, while the proteins will remain trapped inside (fig. 7.2). Small molecules will stop diffusing from inside the tubing when their concentration reaches equilibrium on both sides of the membrane. By changing the buffer solution several times, most of the small molecules can be removed from the extract.

Materials for Part B:

☐ tissue extract
☐ 12 inches dialysis tubing (12,000–14,000 MW exclusion limit)
☐ 2 tubing clamps
☐ 2 50-ml tubes
☐ 5 liters saline solution
☐ magnetic stir bar and stir plate
☐ 2-liter flask
☐ Pasteur pipettes
☐ refrigerator
☐ clinical centrifuge

Procedure:

1. Cut an approximately 12-inch length of dialysis tubing. Soak it in a beaker of distilled water about 10 minutes, then rinse it in 3 changes of distilled water.

2. Clamp one end of the tubing shut, being careful not to stretch the tubing and possibly enlarge the pores. Using a Pasteur pipette, place the tissue extract into the tubing, leaving a 1/2-inch head space. Clamp the top shut.

3. Place the filled tubing in a large flask containing 1 liter of saline and a magnetic stir bar. Stir gently at 4°C.

4. Change the saline solution 4 times over a period of 2 to 4 days.

5. After the dialysis is complete, carefully unclamp one end of the tubing and transfer the protein to a 50-ml tube. If there is debris or precipitate present in the protein solution, centrifuge the solution at $1800 \times g$ for 15 minutes and transfer the supernatant to a new tube. Discard the debris.

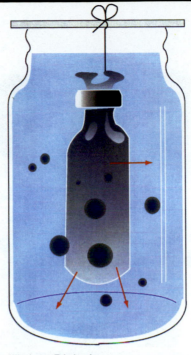

Figure 7.2   Equilibrium Dialysis

C.   Calculation of Protein Concentration

It will be necessary to know the concentration of the protein in order to use it for immunization. There are many colorimetric procedures for determining protein concentration, but the following is a particularly simple and rapid method using the protein-binding dye Coomassie Blue. This dye undergoes a color change from brown to blue after binding to protein (fig. 7.3). The amount of blue color can be determined spectrophotometrically by absorbance at a wavelength of 595 nm. If the dye is added to a set of protein standards of known concentration, a standard curve can be constructed by plotting the absorbance reading (optical density) versus protein concentration. The concentration of your tissue protein sample can then be derived by measuring its absorbance and extrapolating the concentration from the standard curve. It is important that the absorbance reading for the unknown sample (the tissue protein) fall within the range of the standard curve, and below a reading of 1.0 O. D. If your sample is too concentrated, you will have to prepare several dilutions of the original sample to find one that falls within the curve.

Materials for Part C:

- ☐ 100 mls Bio-Rad™ protein assay reagent (contains Coomassie Blue)
- ☐ 1 ml standard protein solution (bovine or porcine albumin, 2.0 mg/ml in saline)
- ☐ 25 mls saline solution
- ☐ test tubes (about 30)
- ☐ 1-ml pipettes (about 30)
- ☐ spectrophotometer (visible range)
- ☐ sterile filtration unit

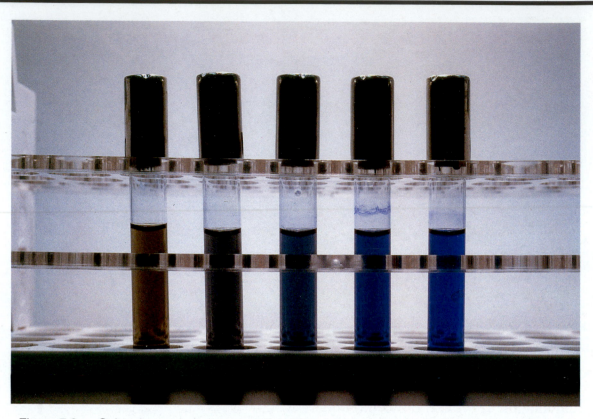

Figure 7.3   Color change between samples of increasing protein concentration in the Bio-Rad

Procedure:

1. Prepare eight two-fold dilutions of the standard protein in 0.5 mls saline (fig. 7.4). Calculate the actual protein concentration of each dilution (starting concentration is 2 mg/ml).

2. Your tissue protein sample will probably be too concentrated, so also prepare three or four ten-fold dilutions of the sample in saline.

3. *Do not* add the Bio-Rad dye reagent directly to your dilutions. Transfer 0.1 ml from each dilution of the standard and the sample to a new, labeled tube. Also place 0.1 mls saline in a tube labeled "blank."

4. Add 5.0 mls of the Bio-Rad reagent to each of the new tubes, including the blank. Mix the tubes, then let sit for 5 minutes (or up to 1 hour).

5. Use your "blank" to adjust the spectrophotometer to zero absorbance, then measure the absorbance of each tube. Find the dilution of your tissue protein sample which best fits within the standard curve range. It may be necessary to make more ten-fold dilutions, or to make additional dilutions which fall in between if the ten-fold increment is too large.

6. Plot the absorbance values of the standard dilutions versus concentration (in mg/ml) on linear graph paper. Plot the curve as actual absorbance reading versus protein concentration rather than a line of best fit. Proteins will not show a linear relationship at higher concentrations, as you may notice from your curve. Albumin is chosen as a standard because this is one of the major proteins in your tissue extract. Read the concen-

tration of your tissue protein sample from the curve. If a dilution of the sample was measured, be sure to multiply the concentration by the dilution factor to get the concentration of protein in the original sample.

7. Filter-sterilize the protein solution and either prepare for immunization or store as instructed in experiment 9.

Key Terms:
immunogenic
hapten
carrier protein
equilibrium dialysis
semipermeable membrane

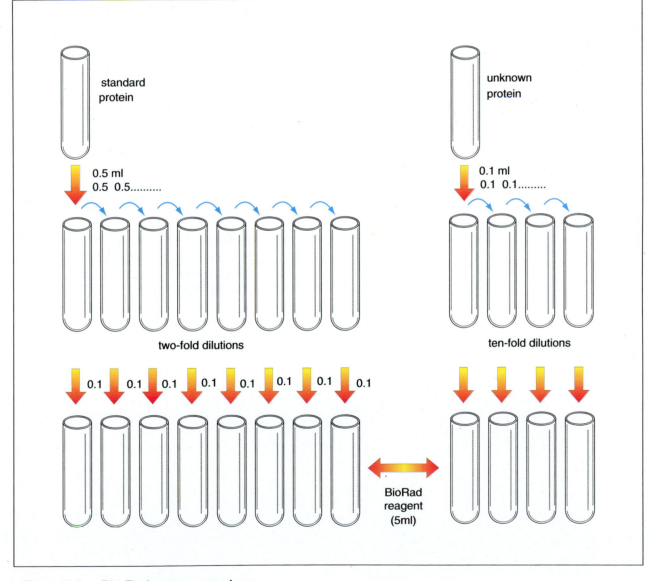

Figure 7.4   Bio-Rad assay procedure

Questions:

1. What is the purpose of the dialysis tubing used in the preparation of the tissue extract?

2. How will your protein antigen be stored after preparation? Why is it stored this way?

3. What features would a highly antigenic molecule have?

Additional Reading:

1. Coligan, J. E., et al., eds. 1991. Current Protocols in Immunology. Greene Publishing Associates and Wiley-Interscience.

2. Garvey, J. S., et al. 1977. Methods in Immunology. A Laboratory Text for Instruction and Research. Reading, Massachusetts: Benjamin/Cummings. Pp. 347–374.

3. McClain, B. R. 1990. Meet the T-cell antigen receptor. The American Biology Teacher 52(5):276–279.

4. Grey, H. M., A. Sette, and S. Buus. 1989. How T-cells see antigen. Sci. Am. 261(5):56.

5. Johnson, H. M., J. K. Russell, and C. H. Pontzer. 1992. Superantigens in human disease. Sci. Am. 266(4):92.

6. Sela, M. 1969. Antigenicity: some molecular aspects. Science 166:1365–1374.

7. Wilson, I. A., H. L. Niman, R. A. Houghten, et al. 1984. The structure of an antigenic determinant in a protein. Cell 37:767–778.

8 Preparation of Cells as Antigens

In exercise 7 you learned how to prepare protein antigens for immunization. Whole cells can also be used to immunize animals directly. Cells are complex antigens with many antigenic sites on their surfaces, and can be administered without the use of an adjuvant. Many vaccines are actually preparations of whole bacteria which have either been killed or modified. In this exercise you will learn how to prepare bacterial and erythrocyte antigens. These antigen preparations can be used for immunization or for agglutination assays.

⚠ **Safety Tips:**
Salmonella species are pathogens. Use caution when handling the culture to avoid splattering, aerosolization, or contamination of hands or face. Wash hands as soon as you are finished handling the culture.

A.   Preparation of Bacterial O Antigens

Gram negative bacteria possess somatic antigens (O antigens) which are important determinants of strain specificities. The O antigens are part of the lipopolysaccharide layer of the gram-negative cell wall. Motile strains of gram-negative bacteria also possess flagellar antigens (H antigens) which must be inactivated before preparing O antigen. The flagellar antigens are heat-labile and can be inactivated by boiling the culture.

Materials for Part A:
- ☐ overnight nutrient broth culture of a *Salmonella* species
- ☐ 1 sterile screw-cap tube
- ☐ 10 mls of sterile saline containing 0.6% formalin
- ☐ McFarland standards
- ☐ 1 tube of thioglycollate broth

- ☐ 60°C water bath
- ☐ clinical centrifuge

Procedure:

Broth cultures are to be prepared the day prior to starting the experiment.

1. Place 5 mls of the broth culture in a glass screw-cap tube. Place the tube in a 60°C water bath for one hour. Make sure the cap on the tube is loosened.

2. Remove the tube from the water bath, and transfer the culture to a 15-ml centrifuge tube. Centrifuge at 1800 × g for 15 minutes in a clinical centrifuge.

3. Decant the supernatant into the discard container, being careful to avoid dripping down the outside of the tube.

4. Resuspend the bacterial pellet in 5 mls of the saline/formalin.

5. Compare the turbidity of the bacterial suspension to McFarland standards number 3 and 4 (see Appendix 3, p. 194). Add saline/formalin to the bacteria to obtain a cell density of approximately 1×10^9 (between the McFarland 3 and 4 standards). It may be necessary to dilute the bacteria several times.

6. Make sure that the bacteria are killed by placing a couple drops of the suspension in a tube of thioglycollate broth and incubating at 37°C. Check the tube for growth after two or three days.

B. Preparation of Bacterial H Antigens

To prepare H antigens, it is necessary to obtain a motile strain of a bacterium. Bacteria may lose their motility after repeated subculturing on solid plate media, so motility must first be enhanced by passage of the bacteria through semi-solid motility medium. The H antigen is then prepared by adding formalin to the motile culture. Formalin fixes the proteins of the flagella so that they are not as labile, and also causes the flagella to extend out from the surface of the cells.

Materials for Part B:

- ☐ overnight nutrient broth culture of a Salmonella species
- ☐ 3 tubes of semi-solid motility medium
- ☐ 5 mls sterile nutrient broth in a large tube that will hold 10 mls
- ☐ 5 mls of sterile saline containing 0.6% formalin
- ☐ 1 sterile screw-cap tube
- ☐ 10 mls sterile saline
- ☐ McFarland standards
- ☐ 1 tube of thioglycollate broth
- ☐ 37°C water bath

Procedure:

1. Prior to preparation of the H antigen, pass the culture through 3 sequential tubes of semi-solid motility medium. This may be done by stabbing down into the tube of motility medium with a loopful of the culture. Incubate the tube at 37°C for one or two days, then transfer some bacteria from the first motility tube to the second in the same manner. Repeat once more with the third tube.

2. Transfer some of the bacteria from the third motility tube to a tube containing nutrient broth. Incubate overnight at 37°C.

3. Add 5 mls saline/formalin to the culture and let stand at room temperature for two to five days.

4. Adjust the bacterial concentration to 1×10^9 cells/ml and check for sterility as in steps 5 and 6 of part A.

C. Preparation of Erythrocyte Antigens

Erythrocytes from any species can be prepared very easily by simply washing the cells in saline prior to use. Whole blood contains about 20% erythrocytes. The concentration of erythrocytes used for immunization is usually 10%, while the concentration used in some of the assays in later exercises is 1 or 2%.

Materials for Part C:

- ☐ 3 to 5 mls sheep blood in Alsever's solution (a preservative)
- ☐ 3 to 5 mls saline
- ☐ 15-ml centrifuge tube
- ☐ clinical centrifuge tube

Procedure:

1. Add the sheep blood to a centrifuge tube, and then add an equal volume of saline.

2. Centrifuge the blood/saline at 800 × g for 10 minutes in a clinical centrifuge.

3. Carefully remove the supernatant with a pipette. The cells will not form a hard pellet and can easily be resuspended if you shake them.

4. Add saline again to double the original volume of the blood.

5. Centrifuge at 800 × g for 10 minutes.

6. Repeat steps 3–5 two more times. After the last centrifugation, remove the supernatant and resuspend the cells in saline to double the original volume of blood to obtain a 10% solution. This suspension may be stored for up to 3 to 4 days at 4°C.

Questions:

1. Why is it usually not necessary to mix antigen composed of whole cells with an adjuvant prior to immunization?

2. Can you name a human vaccine composed of killed microorganisms? What about a human vaccine composed of modified live microorganisms?

Additional Reading:

1. Edwards, P. R., and W. H Ewing. 1972. Identification of Enterobacteriaceae. 3rd ed. Minneapolis, Minnesota: Burgess Publishing Co.

2. Garvey, J. S., N. E. Cremer, and D. H. Sussdorf. 1977. Methods in Immunology. 3rd ed. Reading, Massachusetts: Benjamin/Cummings.

9 Antibody Production in the Rabbit

Many immunological procedures require the use of antibody directed against a specific antigen. An **antiserum** can be produced by injecting an experimental animal with the desired antigen to stimulate **humoral immunity**. The antigen will first be "processed" by macrophages, and then "presented" by the macrophages to B-cell lymphocytes (fig. 9.1). The B-cells have surface-bound antibody which reacts to a particular epitope on the antigen. With the help of certain chemical signals from the T-cell lymphocytes, the B-cells differentiate into immunoglobulin-secreting cells (plasma cells). Within a few weeks the animal will begin producing detectable antibody, which can be harvested in the blood serum. This process is termed **immunization**. **Vaccination** is the term usually reserved for animals or humans being immunized to prevent disease, where the antigen is either a weakened (attenuated) or killed microorganism, or a protein derived from a pathogenic microorganism.

Most useful antigens are complex macromolecules which contain a variety of antigenic sites (epitopes). The antiserum an animal produces in response to large antigens usually consists of a heterogeneous mixture of antibodies of differing epitope specificity and binding affinity. Such an antiserum may be crossreactive with other, similar macromolecules. Other procedures are required if antibody of only a single specificity is desired.

This experiment will require several weeks to complete, and will proceed according to the following outline of activities.

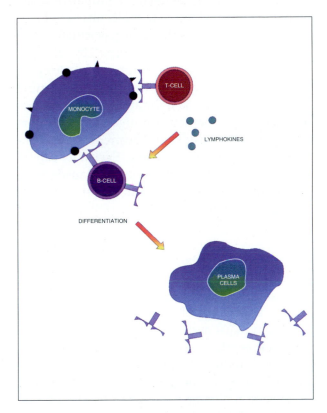

Figure 9.1   Presentation of antigen to the B cell by the macrophage

1. Prepare an antigen for immunization.

2. Immunize and boost the rabbit with the antigen.

3. Monitor the rabbit's serum for production of antibody by the Ascoli test.

4. Demonstrate the specificity of the antibody by Ouchterlony and ELISA.

Part 1. Selection of Antigens and Experimental Animals

The immunization process requires information regarding both the antigen to be used and the animal species selected. For example, it is necessary to know whether the antigen is a protein or a carbohydrate, of small or large molecular weight, in pure or crude form, soluble or particulate, or in readily available or limited supply. In selecting the animal species, the volume of antiserum needed, the availability, health, and immune status of the animal, and the ability of that species to respond to a particular antigen are all factors which must be considered. The preparation of antiserum is not an exact science. Even after careful selections of antigens and animals are made, variable results can be expected due to the inherent biological differences between individuals in a species.

Goats, sheep, and horses are frequently used to produce large volumes of antiserum in industry. Mice are often used when it is desirable to have precise knowledge of the animal's genetic background or to use specially inbred strains. The rabbit is perhaps the most popular species for routine antibody production for research because it requires little space for the relatively large volume of antiserum obtained, is easy to handle, and responds well to a variety of antigens.

Part 2: Preparation of Protein Antigen for Immunization

Antisera to proteins can be prepared by repeated intravenous injections of protein in solution, or by injection of soluble protein emulsified in an adjuvant. Adjuvants are substances which enhance the immune response to an antigen. They are thought to act by making the antigen more insoluble, thus holding the antigen in a localized area (depot) and releasing it slowly over a long period of time. Otherwise, the body would clear the antigen from the circulation very quickly. When immunizing an animal, the *number* of exposures over time to antigen is more important than the size of the antigen dose. Repeat exposures to an antigen result in a secondary antibody response, which is much larger and longer lasting than the primary response to the first antigen exposure (fig. 9.2). Only 100 μg of protein antigen is required to elicit antibody in the rabbit.

In this experiment, either of two popular adjuvants may be used: Freund's adjuvant, or aluminum hydroxide (Imject™ Alum). **Complete Freund's Adjuvant** (CFA) contains three ingredients: Arlacel A (mannide monooleate—an emulsifying agent); Bayol F (paraffin oil); and killed *Mycobacterium tuberculosis*, a bacterium which adds to the benefits of the adjuvant by stimulating the cellular immune response. CFA is used for the primary (first) immunization. **Incomplete Freund's Adjuvant** (IFA), which lacks the *Mycobacterium* component, is used for secondary (booster) immunizations because the *Mycobacterium* causes a severe hypersensitivity reaction if injected more than once. It is important that the protein antigen be free of contaminants which could alter the immune response. This is achieved by filter sterilization of the protein before mixing with adjuvant.

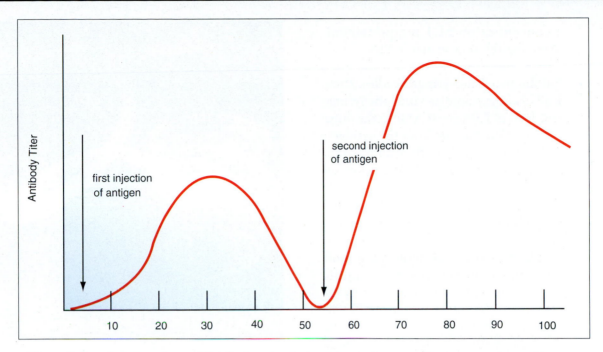

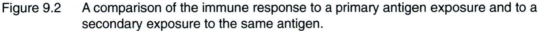

Figure 9.2   A comparison of the immune response to a primary antigen exposure and to a secondary exposure to the same antigen.

A.   Freund's Adjuvant Procedure

Materials for Part A:

- ☐ 2 ml Complete Freund's Adjuvant (or IFA if preparing a booster)
- ☐ protein antigen solution in phosphate buffered saline
- ☐ sterile, cotton-plugged 1-ml pipettes
- ☐ phoshate buffered saline (PBS)
- ☐ membrane filter unit fitted with a 0.45 μm membrane filter
- ☐ 1 large, sterile, capped test tube
- ☐ 2 21-gauge syringe needles and a 10-inch length of polyethylene tubing
- ☐ (0.86 mm ID) or a double-hubbed needle
- ☐ 2 3-ml luer-lock syringes
- ☐ plastic cryotubes
- ☐ 1 beaker containing saline
- ☐ labeling tape
- ☐ blood agar plate and inoculating wire
- ☐ 37°C incubator (optional)

> ⚠ **Safety Tips:**
> **The Freund's complete adjuvant mixture can cause an inflammatory reaction if accidentally inoculated. Do not splatter into the eyes—wear goggles during use.**

Procedure:

1. Unwrap the sterile filter unit, and attach to a vacuum source (fig. 9.3).

2. Pour the antigen solution into the upper cup of the filter unit. While holding the filter unit steady, carefully turn on the vacuum.

3. After filtering all the antigen solution, pour the solution into a large sterile test tube.

4. Based on your Bio-Rad calculations of the concentration of your antigen solution, dilute enough of the antigen solution to prepare 1 ml of working solution having

a concentration of 1 mg protein/ml. Make the dilution in sterile PBS.

5. Fill the two 3-ml syringe needles. Draw 1 ml of antigen solution into one syringe and 1 ml of CFA (or IFA) into the other syringe. Expel all air from the syringes, and connect them with a double-hub syringe needle (fig. 9.4). Make sure all the connections are as tight as possible as a great deal of pressure will be exerted through the syringes.

6. Divide the remaining sterile antigen filtrate into 1-ml aliquots in cryotubes. Check the sterility of the antigen by inoculating a blood agar plate and incubating for 48 hours at 37°C. Label the cryotubes with your name, the name of the antigen, the date, and "filter-sterilized." Store these tubes in the freezer for later use as boosters.

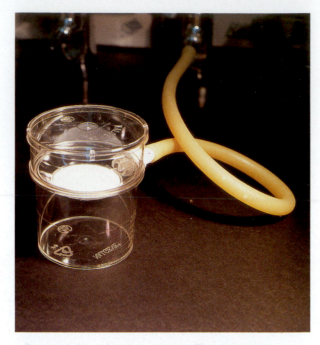

Figure 9.3   Sterile vacuum filtration unit

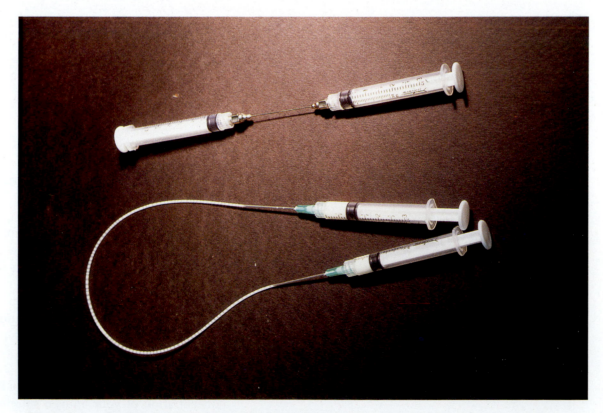

Figure 9.4   Double-hub syringe needle or syringes connected by tubing may be used for preparation of antigen in Freund's adjuvant

7. You will now prepare a "water-in-oil" emulsion. Begin by pushing all the antigen solution slowly into the CFA-containing syringe. Continue pushing the mixture back and forth through the syringes until a *complete emulsion* is formed. This will require a bit of time and a lot of "elbow grease." The emulsion is complete when the following conditions have been met:

- the color is chalky-white

- the emulsion is so stiff that you cannot move it through the syringe, and it is of even stiffness throughout

- after disengaging one syringe, a drop of the emulsion placed on the surface of a beaker of water holds together and does not disperse (fig. 9.5).

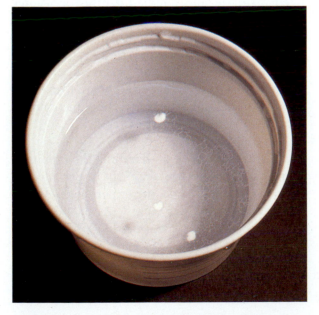

Figure 9.5   Water test of Freund's adjuvant emulsion

8. It is imperative that the emulsion be complete before immunizing the rabbit. It is far better to expend some energy at this point than to have wasted your time when at the end of the semester your rabbit has not produced antibody. Have the instructor check the emulsion when you think it is ready.

   If you get tired, the entire syringe unit may be labeled and placed in the refrigerator (do not freeze!) to work on again later. The mixture may separate somewhat during storage and must be re-emulsified before use. The mixture may be stored refrigerated up to 3 weeks.

9. The antigen/CFA mixture is injected subcutaneously. Booster immunizations may be given every 4 weeks following the primary immunization. Test for antibody production beginning 3 to 4 weeks following the primary immunization and 7 to 10 days after each booster until a high antibody titer is obtained. Once a high titer is reached, it will remain high for some time, allowing the animal to be bled repeatedly to harvest antiserum. Monitor the rabbit's titer with the Ascoli ring test (procedure will be demonstrated in a later exercise).

B.   Alum Adjuvant Procedure

Materials for Part B:

- ☐ 1 ml Imject™ Alum adjuvant
- ☐ protein antigen solution in phosphate buffered saline
- ☐ sterile, cotton-plugged 1-ml pipettes
- ☐ phosphate buffered saline
- ☐ membrane filter unit fitted with a 0.45 mm membrane filter
- ☐ 1 large, sterile, capped test tube
- ☐ small, sterile beaker containing a sterile magnetic stir bar
- ☐ magnetic stir plate
- ☐ plastic cryotubes
- ☐ blood agar plate and inoculating loop
- ☐ 37°C incubator (optional)

Procedure:

1. Unwrap the sterile filter unit, and attach to a vacuum source (fig. 9.3).

2. Pour the antigen solution into the upper cup of the filter unit. While holding the filter unit steady, carefully turn on the vacuum.

3. After filtering all the antigen solution, pour the solution into a large sterile test tube.

4. Based on your Bio-Rad calculations of the concentration of your antigen solution, dilute enough of the antigen solution to prepare 1 ml of working solution having a concentration of 1 mg protein/ ml. Make the dilution in sterile saline.

5. Place the 1 ml of working solution of antigen in a small beaker. Add 1 ml of the Alum solution dropwise to the antigen while stirring. Continue stirring the mixture for 30 minutes.

6. Divide the remaining sterile antigen filtrate into 1-ml aliquots in cryotubes. Check the sterility of the antigen by inoculating a blood agar plate and incubating for 48 hours at 37°C. Label the cryotubes with your name, the name of the antigen, the date, and "filter-sterilized." Store these tubes in the freezer for later use as boosters.

7. The antigen/Alum mixture is injected subcutaneously. Booster immunizations may be given every 4 weeks following the primary immunization. Test for antibody production beginning 3 to 4 weeks following the primary immunization and 7 to 10 days after each booster until a high antibody titer is obtained. Once a high titer is reached, it will remain high for some time, allowing the animal to be bled repeatedly to harvest antiserum. Monitor the rabbit's titer with the Ascoli ring test (procedure will be demonstrated in a later exercise).

Part 3.   Injection and Bleeding of Rabbits

A.   General Care and Handling.

Rabbits usually are mild-tempered animals but are strong enough to inflict serious injury on their handler or themselves when panicked. Therefore, caution must be exercised when picking rabbits up and carrying them around. Your instructor will demonstrate proper methods of carrying and handling rabbits. Remember that the rabbits must be handled as humanely as possible at all times. Report to your instructor any signs of ill health.

Young rabbits (New Zealand or Dutch White) that weigh at least 2.5 kg (5 1/2 lbs) are best for immunization. During experimentation they must be housed correctly, kept clean, fed and watered regularly, and handled gently (occasional vegetarian treats from home are permissible and probably welcomed). Laboratory workers shouldn't forget the importance of properly cared-for animals. All the precise assays and equipment used in an experiment are to no avail if variation of animals used in the same study is not minimized by proper treatment.

It is a good idea to begin handling the rabbits as soon as possible so that they will be accustomed to you when you begin the experiment. All experimental procedures conducted on the rabbit (injections, bleedings, and the like), must be recorded on the animals cage card, and in table 9.1 below.

Table 9.1   Immunization Schedule

Antigen	Date	Amount Injected	Route of Injection

B.   Injection Procedure (Subcutaneous)

Always obtain a sample of normal (naive) serum to use as a control before the primary immunization. All antigen substances, needles, and syringes for injection should be free of contaminating organisms.

Materials for Part B:
- ☐ bottle of 70% ethanol
- ☐ cotton balls
- ☐ antigen in syringe with 21-gauge needle

Procedure:

1. Have another person hold the rabbit down on a hard, slippery surface. Cleanse the injection site with alcohol. Prepare a syringe fitted with a 21-gauge needle containing the antigen/adjuvant mixture.

2. Raise a "tent" of skin on the back of the rabbit's neck with the thumb and index finger of your left hand. Pull the loose skin up away from the rabbit's body (fig. 9.6).

3. With your right hand, insert the *entire* needle through the skin at the front of the "tent," making sure the needle is all the way through and lies under the skin. You will be able to feel the needle "pop" through the skin layer. Keep the needle parallel to the rabbit's body to avoid jabbing the underlying muscle.

4. Inject 0.2 ml of the antigen/adjuvant mixture and withdraw the needle. Inject four other sites around the rabbit's neck, being careful not to inject more than 0.2 ml at one site. Dispose of the needle and syringe in a needle disposal box.

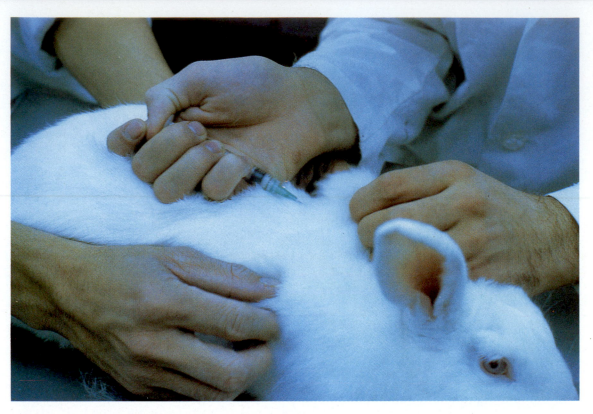

Figure 9.6   Subcutaneous injection of the rabbit

C.   Bleeding Rabbits for Collection of Serum
Materials for Part C:

☐ rabbit restraining box
☐ lamp (with goose neck or movable head that can be directed up through rabbit's ear from below)
☐ blood collection tubes (glass only)
☐ 20-gauge vacutainer needles
☐ cotton balls
☐ bottle of 70% ethanol
☐ large paper clip
☐ clinical centrifuge

Procedure:

1. Place the rabbit in a restraining box and secure so that the animal is too snug to move but not uncomfortable. Allow the rabbit to relax for a few minutes. Meanwhile, have on hand a blood collection tube, a 20-gauge vacutainer needle, several large cotton balls, and a large paper clip.

2. To dilate the blood vessels in the ear, hold the ear over a warm lamp for several minutes (test with your hand to make sure you are not burning the rabbit's skin). It is very important to make sure the vessels are well dilated or you will have difficulty maintaining the blood flow (fig. 9.7A).

3. Shine a small lamp up through the ear to help locate the arterial blood vessel which runs down the center of the ear. Uncover both ends of the vacutainer needle and hold the needle almost parallel (5°) to the ear. Carefully insert the needle into the blood vessel while lowering to a parallel position. You should insert the needle about 1/4 inch into the vessel. The blood will flow out the other end of the needle and can be collected in a tube (fig. 9.7B)

Up to 50 ml can be collected by this method for harvesting antiserum, although it is only necessary to collect 5 to 10 mls of blood for checking the serum titer. If the blood flow stops before you have collected enough, try rubbing the vessel or flicking the ear with your finger with the needle left in place. Be careful not to move the needle around in the blood vessel after inserting it, because it may poke through the wall of the vessel and cause bruising of the ear.

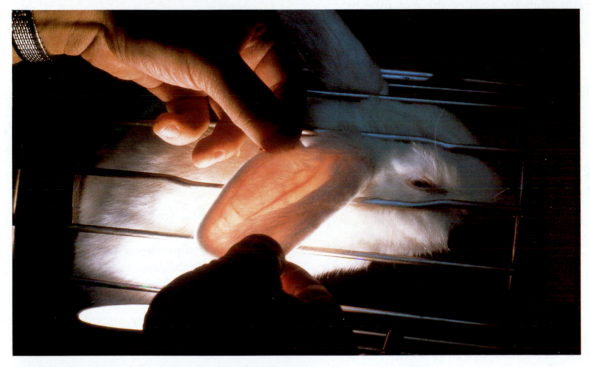

Figure 9.7**A**. Dilation of the blood vessels in the ear over a warm light.

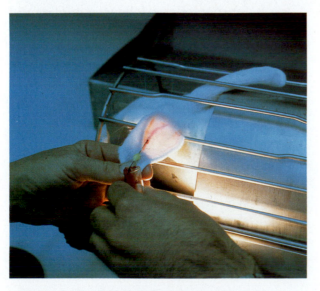

Figure 9.7**B**. Blood samples are drawn from the central artery of the ear using a vacutainer needle.

4. Gently remove the needle and hold a large cotton ball over the insertion site. Place another cotton ball on the opposite side of the ear and hold both in place with a large paper clip. Be sure to remove the paper clip after about 10 minutes!

5. If the bleeding has stopped wash any dried blood from the ear with water. Make *sure* the bleeding has completely stopped before returning the rabbit to the cage. Dispose of the needles in a needle disposal box.

D. Separation and Storage of Serum

1. Allow freshly collected blood to stand at room temperature for clot formation.

2. After 30 minutes, carefully separate the clot from the wall of the test tube by sliding a wooden applicator stick around the inner wall of the tube (rather like loosening a cake from the pan).

3. Place the tube of blood in the refrigerator overnight or up to 48 hours. The clot will contract and squeeze out the serum.

4. Decant the serum (yellowish fluid) into a centrifuge tube. Centrifuge at 1000 × g for 10 minutes to sediment any erythrocytes present in the serum.

5. With a Pasteur pipette, transfer the serum to a storage tube for freezing. Hold the pipette tip just below the top of the fluid to avoid stirring up the pelleted erythrocytes.

6. Store the serum frozen at -20°C.

Key Terms:

serum
antiserum
immunoglobulin
immunization
vaccination
hapten
epitope
immunogen
carrier protein
adjuvant
humoral immunity

Questions:

1. What is the difference between humoral immunity and cellular immunity?

2. How did the term **vaccination** originate?

3. How do adjuvants work? What would happen to the protein antigen if injected without an adjuvant?

4. Why is it necessary to give your rabbit booster immunizations?

5. Graph the change in antibody concentration in the serum of an animal as a function of time following primary and secondary immunization.

6. How would you design an experiment to prove that use of Freund's adjuvant increases antibody production?

7. What are the cellular components required to generate an antibody response and how do they interact?

8. Why is the immune response to an antigen usually heterogenous?

Additional Reading:

Immunization:

1. Freund, J. 1947. Some aspects of active immunization. Ann. Rev. Microbiol. 1:291

2. Freund, J. 1951. The effect of paraffin oil and mycobacteria on antibody formation and sensitization. Am. J. Clin. Pathol. 21:645

3. Behbeham, A. M. 1983. The smallpox story: life and death of an old disease. Microbiological Reviews 47:455–509

4. Lerner, R. A. 1983. Synthetic vaccines. Sci. Am. 248(2):66.

5. Allison, C. A. 1979. Mode of action of immunological adjuvants. J. Res. 26: 619–630.

6. Gregoriadis, G. 1990. Immunological adjuvants: a role for liposomes. Immunol. Today 11(3):89.

7. Moss, B. 1985. Vaccinia virus expression vector: a new tool for immunologists. Immunol. Today 6:243–245.

The Antibody Response:

1. Edelman, G. M. 1970. The structure and function of antibodies. Sci. Am. 223(2):34–42.

2. Grey, H. M., and R. Chesnut. 1985. Antigen processing and presentation to T cells. Immunol. Today 6:101–106.

3. Smith, K. A. 1990. Interleukin-2. Sci. Am. 262(3):50.

4. Miedema, F., and C. J. M. Melief. 1983. T cell regulation of human B cell activation. Immunol. Today 6:258–259.

5. Unanue, E. R. 1980. Cooperation between mononuclear phagocytes and lymphocytes in immunity. N. Engl. J. Med. 303:977–985.

Use of Laboratory Animals:

1. Tuffery, B. R. 1987. Lab Animals: An Introduction for New Experimenters. Chichester, England: John Wiley and Sons.

2. U. S. Dept. of Health and Human Services. 1985. Guide for the Care and Use of Laboratory Animals. ILAR Committee on the Care and Use of Laboratory Animals. NIH Pub. No. 86–23. Washington, D. C. (free publication).

10 Transfer of Humoral Immunity -- Passive Immunization

In exercise 9 a rabbit was injected with an antigen in order to generate an antibody response. This process is called "active immunization." In humans, as in rabbits, active immunization occurs either artificially when you are vaccinated against disease or naturally when you acquire an infection like a cold or the chicken pox. In either case, your own immune mechanisms are stimulated to produce the antibodies that will give you long-lasting protection against the specific infectious agent.

Protection from disease can also be conferred when serum from an individual who already has antibodies is transferred to an individual who doesn't. This type of protection is termed "passive immunization," and is short-lived because the antibodies will eventually be catabolized. An example of naturally ocurring passive immunization is the transfer of antibody across the placenta from the mother to the fetus. At birth, an infant is protected from any pathogen that the mother is immune to. This protection lasts about 6 months; about the time that babies begin producing their own antibody responses to any infectious agents that they encounter. Antibody can also be transferred through the breast milk to the nursing infant.

Another example of passive transfer of immunity is the administration of antibody against the tetanus toxin to patients who have been exposed to the *Clostridium tetani* bacterium but were never vaccinated. In the early days of such treatment, the tetanus antibody was prepared by immuniz-

ing horses with formaldehyde-inactivated tetanus toxin (tetanus toxoid). The toxoid is rendered non-toxic by this treatment but remains immunogenic. The serum from these horses was then given to patients. Unfortunately, patients who were given horse serum often suffered severe hypersensitivity reactions because their immune systems reacted to the foreign horse serum proteins. Now, human anti-tetanus serum is available for patient treatment. There are several other diseases which can be treated by passive immunization, including diphtheria, rabies, botulism, and type B hepatitis.

The following simple exercise will demonstrate how the passive transfer of antibody can protect mice from *Streptococcus pneumoniae*, an organism to which mice are extremely susceptible.

Materials:

- [ ] 2 mice
- [ ] 0.5 mls *Streptococcus pneumoniae* antiserum
- [ ] 0.5 mls normal serum
- [ ] 2 mls *Streptococcus pneumoniae* broth culture, incubated
- [ ] overnight and diluted 1:10,000 in sterile saline
- [ ] 2 different colored markers for marking mice
- [ ] 4 1-ml syringes with 25-gauge needles
- [ ] 70% ethanol and cotton balls
- [ ] mouse jar with chloroform and cotton balls

61

Procedure:

The broth culture is to be prepared the day prior to starting the exercise.

1. Mark each of the two mice with different colors or keep them in separate cages so that each can be identified later.

2. Inject mouse #1 with 0.5 ml antiserum. Inject mouse #2 with 0.5 ml normal serum. The injections should be intraperitoneal (see exercise 2).

3. After 24 hours, inject both mice with 0.5 ml diluted S. pneumoniae.

4. Check mice daily over a period of 96 hours for signs of illness. Mice that are ill will be lethargic and will have rumpled fur, and may have mucus in the eyes or nose. Euthanize any mice that become ill by placing them in a jar or coffee can containing a couple of large cotton balls that have been soaked in chloroform. Leave mice in the jar for 5 minutes.

Questions:

1. What are the differences between active and passive immunization? Give some examples of each.

2. Why does the immunity you gain from childhood vaccinations usually last a lifetime?

3. Why is formaldehyde used to make vaccines from bacteria or bacterial toxins?

Additional Reading:

1. Berkman, S. A., M. L. Lee, and R. P. Gale. 1990. Clinical uses of intravenous immunoglobulins. Ann Intern. Med. 112:278.

Section 2

Serological Assays

Serology is the study of immune reactions mediated by serum factors such as antibody and complement. There are many different serological assays which utilize the antibody/antigen reaction. These assays are particularly useful in clinical laboratories for the preliminary diagnosis of infection by detection of infectious material in patient specimens and for the confirmation of a diagnosis by demonstration of the presence of specific antibody against the suspected pathogen in the patient's serum. Many of these methods are also used in research laboratories. Several different types of serological assays will be presented in section 2.

11 Agglutination Reactions -- Three Methods

If a suspension of particulate (large, easily sedimented) antigens such as animal cells, erythrocytes, or bacteria is mixed with serum which contains the corresponding antibody, the antigen particles will form visible clumps. This reaction is termed **agglutination** and is caused by the bridging of antigen particles by antibody molecules to form larger aggregates (fig. 11.1). The agglutination reaction is similar to another serological reaction, **precipitation**. The main difference between the two reactions is the size of the antigen. Precipitation is the aggregation of **soluble** antigen (molecular size). Agglutination reactions are usually somewhat more sensitive than precipitation reactions because a smaller soluble antigen must combine with much more antibody than a similar amount of particulate antigen before a visible aggregate is formed. Nevertheless, both reactions are highly specific because they rely on specific antibody. It is possible to make the detection of soluble antigen/antibody aggregates more sensitive by linking soluble antigen to inert particulate carriers such as erythrocytes or latex beads to simulate the agglutination reaction. This application is termed **passive agglutination**.

Serological reactions such as agglutination have many applications in clinical medicine. Among the most familiar are the typing of blood cells for transfusion, the identification of bacterial cultures with known antisera, and the detection of specific antibody in a patient's serum with known cultures of bacteria. For example, if a patient is suspected of having typhoid fever, the patient's serum is mixed with a culture of *Salmonella typhi*.

If clumping of the bacteria occurs, the patient may be assumed to have antibody to *S. typhi*. However, because certain antibody classes (IgG) persist in the serum for years, it would still be uncertain whether the patient is currently suffering from typhoid fever or had the disease some time in the past and is now ill with something else. For this reason, it is customary to test a patient's serum twice to confirm an illness: first at the onset of illness (an "acute" serum), and then again about two weeks later (a "convalescent" serum). If the **titer** (amount) of antibody in the patient's serum has increased at least four-fold between the two samples, it can be assumed the patient is currently fighting off the infection, and illness with the suspected pathogen is confirmed.

In this exercise you will perform several types of agglutination assays. The assays will include the rapid slide test, the tube dilution test, and the microtiter test.

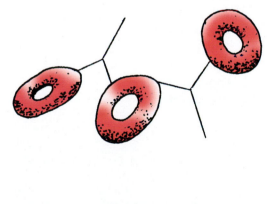

Figure 11.1   Agglutination of erythrocytes

> ⚠ *Safety Tips:*
> 1. **Prick your own finger and handle only your own blood. Do not exchange lancets.**
> 2. **All sharp objects, including pins and lancets, and agglutination slides are to be disposed of in a biohazard container. Under no circumstances are they to be thrown in the trash cans.**
> 3. **Avoid contact with the bacterial antigen preparation and the A, B, D antisera—they should be considered possibly infectious.**

A. Rapid Slide Agglutination

This is a valuable method for rapid detection of an antigen/antibody reaction. Applications of this method include A-B-O blood typing tests (fig. 11.3), pregnancy tests (passive agglutination), and rapid bacterial identification.

You will perform an ABO/Rh blood typing test on your own blood, and a bacterial slide agglutination test.

Materials for Part A:

- ☐ bacterial antigens in dropper bottles (test strain and negative control)
- ☐ anti-bacterial antiserum in a dropper bottle
- ☐ anti-A, B, and D(Rh) antisera in dropper bottles
- ☐ saline in a dropper bottle
- ☐ 2 microscope slides
- ☐ wax pencil
- ☐ lancet (sterile)
- ☐ 70% ethanol or alcohol swab
- ☐ cotton ball
- ☐ fingertip bandage
- ☐ 7 toothpicks

Procedure:

1. With a wax pencil draw three 1" diameter circles on one slide and label the circles A, B, and C for the bacterial test (fig. 11.2). On the other slide draw four 1" circles and label these A–D for the blood typing test.

2. Place one drop of the appropriate *antigen* on the circles of each slide according to figure 11.2. For the blood test you will use a drop of your own blood on each circle as the antigen (see instructions for pricking your finger in Experiment 1, part B).

3. Place one drop of the appropriate antiserum on the circles of each slide according to figure 11.2. Do not contaminate the tip of the droppers with antigen.

4. Mix the drops in each of the circles, using separate toothpicks.

5. Gently rock the slides for two minutes under a bright light. Look for granules or clumping. There should be no agglutination in control circles. Record your results on figure 11.2.

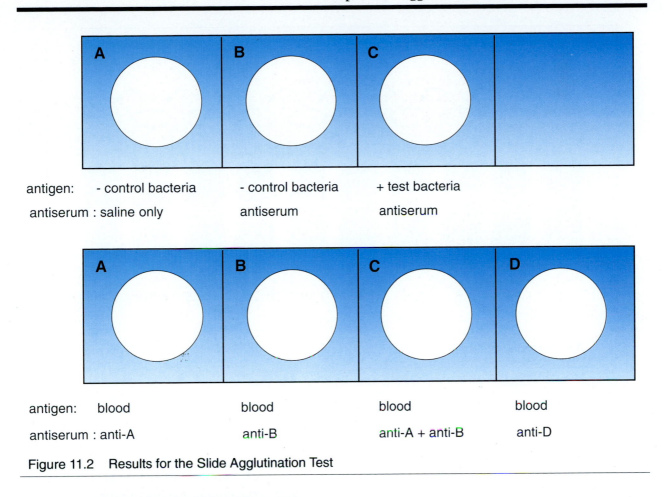

antigen: - control bacteria   - control bacteria   + test bacteria

antiserum : saline only   antiserum   antiserum

antigen: blood   blood   blood   blood

antiserum : anti-A   anti-B   anti-A + anti-B   anti-D

Figure 11.2   Results for the Slide Agglutination Test

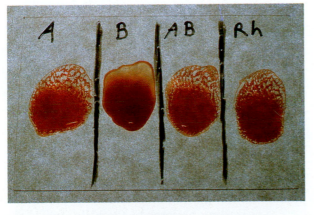

Figure 11.3   Slide agglutination test used in blood typing.

B.   Tube Dilution Test

A tube test for *quantifying* the amount of agglutinating antibodies present in an antiserum was first described in 1896 by Grunbaum and Widal. The "Widal" test for typhoid fever is still in use today, and the procedure has been applied to many other illnesses as well.

Various dilutions of the test antiserum are prepared and these are mixed with a constant amount of antigen. After incubation, the tubes are examined for agglutination. The highest dilution of antiserum (most dilute tube) which still exhibits agglutination is designated the **endpoint dilution**. The reciprocal of the endpoint dilution value is called the antibody **titer**. For example, if two-fold serial dilutions of serum are prepared and the 1:320 dilution is the last tube still containing enough antibody to cause visible agglutination, the patient's titer is expressed as 320 **agglutination units of antibody**.

For this test you will determine the titer of rabbit antiserum against sheep red blood cells.

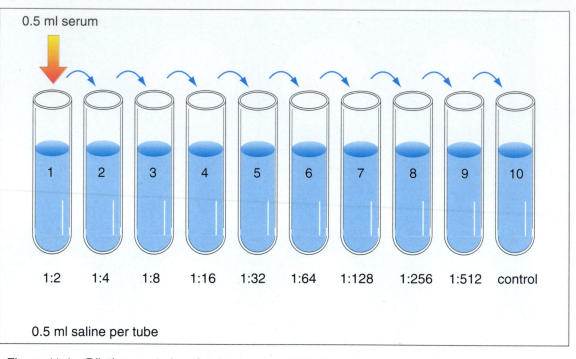

0.5 ml serum

| 1 | 2 | 3 | 4 | 5 | 6 | 7 | 8 | 9 | 10 |

| 1:2 | 1:4 | 1:8 | 1:16 | 1:32 | 1:64 | 1:128 | 1:256 | 1:512 | control |

0.5 ml saline per tube

Figure 11.4   Dilution procedure for the tube agglutination test

Materials for Part B:

☐ 0.5 mls anti-SRBC antiserum (rabbit)
☐ 10 mls SRBC antigen (2% in PBS)
☐ 10 mls normal saline or PBS
☐ 10 test tubes
☐ 2 10-ml sterile pipettes
☐ 20 1-ml sterile pipettes
☐ 37°C water bath

Procedure:

1. Place 10 test tubes in a tube rack. Label the tubes 1 through 10. Tube 10 will be a negative control.

2. Add 0.5 ml saline to every tube with a 10-ml pipette.

3. Add 0.5 ml of the appropriate antiserum to tube 1 with a 1-ml pipette. Mix tube 1 and with a new 1-ml pipette, transfer 0.5 ml from tube 1 to tube 2 (fig. 11.4).

4. Using a new pipette for each transfer, continue transferring 0.5 ml through to tube 9. Mix and discard 0.5 ml from tube 9. Tube 10 will contain no antis-

erum and all the tubes will still contain a total volume of 0.5 ml. You should now have 9 two-fold dilutions of serum (1:2 through 1:512), and a negative control containing only saline.

5. Add 0.5 ml SRBC antigen to all the tubes using a 10-ml pipette.

6. Mix all the tubes by shaking the rack 3 or 4 times. Place the rack in a 37°C water bath for approximately 1–2 hours or incubate overnight at room temperature.

7. To read the results, hold the test tube rack above your head and look up through the bottoms of the tubes at the settling patterns of the cells (fig. 11.5). Agglutination will result in a diffuse layer of cells covering the entire bottom of the test tube because the cells are being bridged apart in a network by antibody molecules. In contrast, cells which do not agglutinate are able to roll down to the very bottom of the tube where they compact into a small pellet. Begin with the negative control so that you

will see what a negative reaction looks like and will be able to recognize agglu-

tination if it occurs. Record your results in table 11.1.

Table 11.1   Tube and Microtiter Agglutination Results

| Dilution of Serum | | | | | | | | | |
Test	1:2	1:4	1:8	1:16	1:32	1:64	1:128	1:256	1:512	control
tubes									,	
micro.									,	

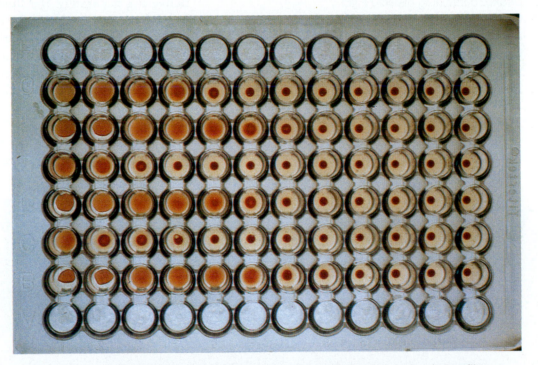

Figure 11.5   Settling pattern of erythrocytes in an agglutination assay (microfilter assay shown here). Cells that agglutinate form a diffuse layer covering the bottom of the well. Cells that do not agglutinate form a compact pellet on the bottom of the well.

Part C: Microtiter Test

Titration in small volumes is often utilized to speed up reaction times and conserve reagents. The procedure was developed in 1955 and is often used for agglutination testing, complement fixation, and neutralization assays. Microtiter plates are plastic disposable trays containing 96 small wells. The wells may have round, conical, or flat bottoms depending on the procedure to be carried out. The special equipment designed for

working with microtiter plates include the "drop-delivery micropipettes" and the "transfer microdiluters" (fig. 11.6). Each drop released by the micropipette is a 50 µl volume. The transfer diluter will pick up, by capillary action, exactly 50 µl and deliver the liquid to the next well. Although the microtiter assay is comparable in sensitivity and reproducibility to the tube test if done correctly, the procedure must be carried out carefully and precisely because smaller volumes are more prone to error. Carry out the following microtiter assay procedure with sheep red blood cells and compare the titers to those obtained from the tube test.

Materials for Part C:

- ☐ 1 microtiter plate and sealing tape
- ☐ 3 micropipettes (50 μl size) and bulb
- ☐ drop delivery micropipettes
- ☐ 1 microdiluter
- ☐ transfer microdiluters
- ☐ cotton swabs
- ☐ beaker containing distilled H₂O
- ☐ beaker containing normal saline or PBS
- ☐ beaker containing 0.5% sodium hypochloride (bleach)
- ☐ blotter paper with calibration circles
- ☐ Bunsen burner

Procedure:

1. Flame the microdiluter in a bunsen burner and allow to cool. This is done once every 20 uses (tests) to remove oxide from the metal surfaces.

2. Test whether you are using the pipetter correctly and whether its delivery is accurate. To do this, wet the diluter in saline contained in a beaker. Make sure the level of the saline does not come above the bevel portion of the diluter head. Diluent that gets on the shaft may roll down and cause inaccurate delivery. Now touch the diluter to the center of a blotter circle. If the diluter is filling and delivering accurately, the fluid should just fill the circle. If not, the diluter is either not properly wetted (try again), or requires calibration. If the diluter is delivering properly, begin the test (diagrammed in figure 11.7).

3. Place the microtiter plate on a damp paper towel. This helps guard against static charges.

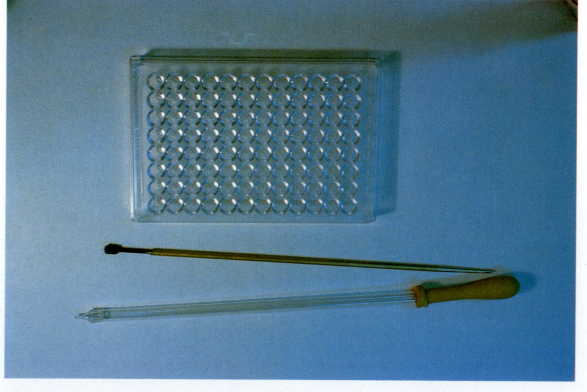

Figure 11.6   Drop delivery micropipette, transfer microdiluter, and microtiter plate.

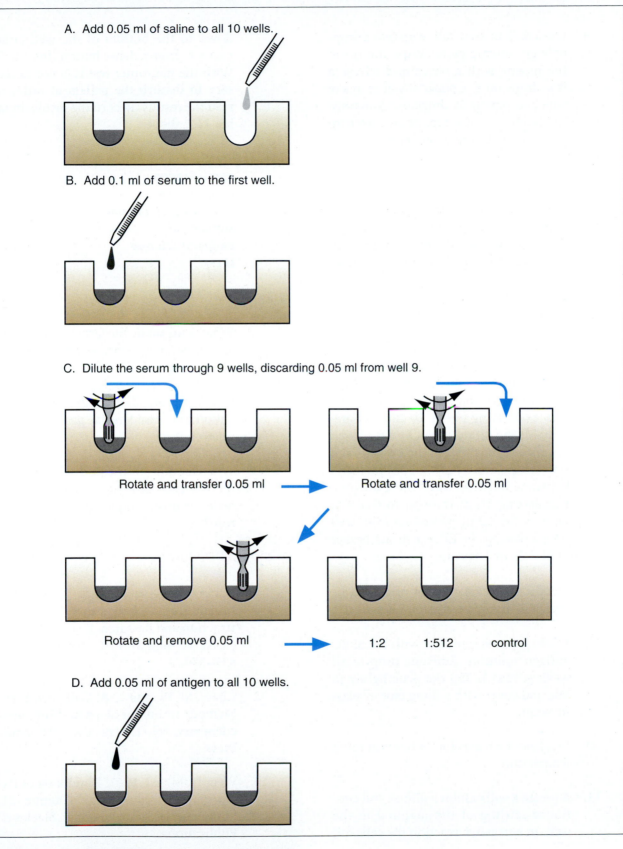

A. Add 0.05 ml of saline to all 10 wells.

B. Add 0.1 ml of serum to the first well.

C. Dilute the serum through 9 wells, discarding 0.05 ml from well 9.

Rotate and transfer 0.05 ml   Rotate and transfer 0.05 ml

Rotate and remove 0.05 ml   1:2   1:512   control

D. Add 0.05 ml of antigen to all 10 wells.

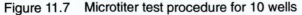

Figure 11.7   Microtiter test procedure for 10 wells

4. Use a bulb to draw saline up into a drop-delivery micropipette. Wipe the tip of the pipette with a tissue and release a few drops onto a paper towel to make sure the pipette is dropping smoothly. Air bubbles in the pipette or a wet tip can cause inaccurate delivery.

5. Holding the pipette exactly vertical, place one drop of saline in all wells of row A of the microtiter plate. If you accidently get more than one drop in a well, remove the diluent from that well with a cotton-tipped swab and try again.

6. Use a micropipette to place one drop of antiserum in the first well.

7. Dip the diluter in the beaker of saline to wet, and blot. Immediately begin making the dilutions in the first row. Place the diluter in the first well (1A), and mix by rotating about 10 times. Carefully lift the diluter straight out of well 1A, picking up 50 µl in the process, and transfer the diluter to well 2A. Mix, and transfer 50 µl to well 3A. Continue transferring 50 µl through to well 9A. Discard the 50 µl picked up from well 9A by placing the diluter in the beaker of bleach for 1 minute.

8. Blot the diluter and rinse by placing in the beaker of distilled water for 1 minute.

9. Fill a clean micropipette with the SRBC antigen solution. Add one drop to all wells of row A. Tap the plate lightly to mix and cover with sealing tape or plastic wrap.

10. Incubate the plates for 24 hours at room temperature.

11. A positive will exhibit a diffuse and confluent settling of the material in the well. In a negative reaction the cells roll down to the bottom of the well compactly to from a dense button (fig. 11.5). With the microtiter test it is not necessary to disturb the pellets in order to read the results. Record the results in table 11.1 above.

Key Terms:

agglutination
precipitation
passive agglutination
serological
endpoint dilution
titer

Questions:

1. What is meant by the terms "sensitivity" and "specificity" when referring to a test procedure?

2. Why is the standard pregnancy agglutination test considered a "passive" agglutination test?

3. What modification could you make in the bacterial slide agglutination test to make results with patient sera easier to read?

Additional Reading:

1. Garvey, J. S., et al. 1977. Methods in Immunology. A Laboratory Text for Instruction and Research. Reading, Massachusetts: Benjamin/Cummings. Pgs. 347–374.

2. Chase, M. W., and C. A. Williams. 1967. Methods in Immunology and Immunochemistry, vol. 1. New York: Academic Press.

3. Weir, D. M., ed. 1967. Handbook of Experimental Immunology. Chapter 21. Philadelphia, Pennsylvania: Blackwell Publications.

Agglutination is the reaction of specific antibody with **particulate** antigen to form large, insoluble aggregates. Even though soluble antigens also form insoluble aggregates with antibody, precipitation reactions are less sensitive because a greater amount of antibody must be combined with the smaller antigens before the aggregates can be detected visually. It is still useful to carry out precipitation reactions in some circumstances, such as when using agarose gels (as you will see in exercise 13), but it is possible to carry out highly sensitive agglutination assays with soluble antigens if either the antigen or the antibody is bound to a larger, insoluble carrier. This technique is called "**passive agglutination.**" Passive agglutination methods using antigen-coated carriers allow the detection of as little as 0.02 mg of antibody in a serum.

Sheep erythrocytes and latex particles are two types of carriers that are widely used. Sheep erythrocytes make good carriers because when treated with a solution of tannic acid, they will readily absorb both polysaccharides and proteins. Erythrocyte carriers do have some disadvantages in that they have a shorter shelf life than latex particles and that there may be crossreactive antibodies in the test serum that react with cellular antigens on the erythrocytes. Therefore, tanned erythrocytes must be prepared fresh, and normal serum must be added to the reaction mixture to inhibit spontaneous agglutination.

Although passive agglutination is an old technique, many current applications exist. An example of passive agglutination used in clinical medicine is the pregnancy test for the presence of human chorionic gonadotropin hormone in the blood or urine. Another example is the test for rheumatoid factor found in the serum of people with rheumatoid arthritis, an autoimmune disease. Rheumatoid factor is antibody produced by the patient against his or her own IgG. In this test, latex particles coated with IgG agglutinate in the presence of patient serum containing rheumatoid factor.

In this exercise, you will prepare antigen-coated erythrocytes using tannic acid, then determine the sensitivity and the specificity of the passive agglutination test system. You will use a microtitration procedure similar to that used in exercise 11.

Materials:

- [ ] 2 mls 10% sheep erythrocytes in PBS
- [ ] 2 mls tannic acid, diluted 1:5000 in PBS (pH 7.2)
- [ ] phosphate buffered saline, (pH 7.2)
- [ ] phosphate buffered saline, (pH 6.4)
- [ ] 1% normal serum in PBS (NRS-PBS)
- [ ] 0.2% sensitizing antigen such as bovine serum albumin (BSA)
- [ ] 0.2% solutions of several other protein antigens (e.g., porcine, sheep, or chicken albumins)
- [ ] test antiserum against the sensitizing antigen, diluted 1:1000 in NRS-PBS
- [ ] clinical centrifuge
- [ ] 15-ml centrifuge tube

Procedure:

A. Procedure for Tanning Sheep Red Blood Cells (SRBC)

1. Add 2 mls of the tannic acid solution to 2 mls of the 10% SRBC in a centrifuge tube. Incubate the mixture for 10 minutes in a 37°C water bath.

2. Centrifuge the SRBC at 500 × g for 5 minutes. Decant the supernatant from the pelleted cells and discard it. Add 15

mls of PBS (pH 7.2) to the pellet and re-suspend the cells to wash them.

3. Centrifuge the SRBC again at $500 \times g$ for 5 minutes, then discard the supernatant as before. Resuspend the tanned cells to a 5% concentration by adding 4 mls of PBS, pH 6.4. The cells are now ready to be coated, or "sensitized" with antigen.

B. Procedure for Sensitization of Tanned Sheep Erythrocytes

1. Set aside 1 ml of 5% tanned SRBC for use as unsensitized control cells. To the remaining 3 mls of tanned SRBC add 3 mls of sensitizing antigen (e.g., BSA). Mix well.

2. Allow the sensitization reaction to take place at room temperature for 30 minutes.

3. Centrifuge the sensitized SRBC at $500 \times g$ for 5 minutes. Discard the supernatant and wash the cells in 15 mls of PBS (pH 6.4).

4. Repeat step 3 above to wash the cells once more.

5. Centrifuge both the sensitized SRBC and the control SRBC you set aside before at $500 \times g$ for 5 minutes. Discard the supernatants and resuspend each pellet to a concentration of 1% by adding 15 mls of the NRS-PBS to the sensitized SRBC and 5 mls NRS-PBS to the control SRBC.

C. Passive Agglutination Procedure

The test antiserum can now be titrated. This test procedure should be performed in duplicate. See part D for the specificity testing procedure. Part D can be carried out at the same time as part C; the only difference is that different antigens are used.

1. To each of the first 11 wells in a 12-well row of a microtiter plate add 50 l of NRS-PBS.

2. To the first well of the row add 50 μl of the diluted antiserum.

3. Prepare 2-fold serial dilutions by transferring 50 μl through the first 10 wells only. Discard 50 μl from the 10th well after mixing. Well 11 is a negative control containing only 50 μl of diluent and no antiserum, to check that the cells can settle correctly if antibody is absent.

4. To each of the first 11 wells add 50 μl of the sensitized SRBC suspension.

5. To the 12th well add 50 μl antiserum and 50 μl of the *control* SRBC.

6. Mix the wells by gently tapping the sides of the microtiter plate. Wrap the plate with plastic wrap and incubate for 60–90 minutes at room temperature.

7. Examine the plate for agglutination against a white background. Determine the titer by observing the settling pattern. Wells 11 and 12 should show no agglutination.

D. Procedure for Testing Specificity

Follow the same procedure as given in part C above with additional rows on the microtiter plate, except using different antigens for each test.

Additional Reading:

1. Boyden, S. V. 1951. The adsorption of proteins on erythrocytes treated with tannic acid and subsequent hemagglutination by anti-protein serum. J. Exp. Med. 93:107.

2. Sever, J. L. 1962. Application of a micro-technique to visual serological investigations. J. Immunol. 88:320.

13 Precipitation Reactions

The precipitation reaction was first described in 1897 by Krause. It is similar to the agglutination reaction studied in the previous exercise in that both are highly specific serological reactions involving the binding of antigen by antibody. The difference between the two reactions lies in the size of the antigen involved. When soluble (molecular size) antigens such as proteins or carbohydrates are bound by antibody to form a cross-linked "lattice" structure, the reaction is called precipitation.

The precipitation reaction is subject to inhibition if either antigen or antibody is present in great excess (figure 13.1). For example, if excess antigen is present, both binding sites of most antibody molecules will be filled with separate antigen molecules so that cross-linking cannot occur. If excess antibody is present, all available antigenic epitopes may be bound by separate antibody molecules, again preventing cross-linking.

Only when antigen and antibody concentrations are optimal, with neither in great excess, will much cross-linking and lattice formation occur. The range of optimal concentration, at which the greatest amount of precipitation occurs, is called the **equivalence zone**.

Assays utilizing the precipitation reaction range from the simple ring test to highly accurate and quantitative methods. These assays have many applications, such as the identification and classification of microorganisms, the detection of specific antibody in the diagnosis of infectious diseases, the quantitative determination of protein concentrations, and the study of antigen and antibody valences, binding site size, and forces involved in binding.

For this exercise, you will perform three assays based on simple diffusion: the Ascoli ring test, the Ouchterlony test, and the Mancini test.

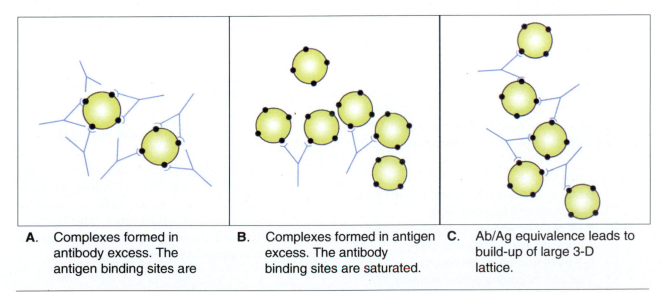

A. Complexes formed in antibody excess. The antigen binding sites are

B. Complexes formed in antigen excess. The antibody binding sites are saturated.

C. Ab/Ag equivalence leads to build-up of large 3-D lattice.

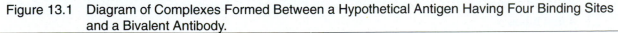

Figure 13.1   Diagram of Complexes Formed Between a Hypothetical Antigen Having Four Binding Sites and a Bivalent Antibody.

75

This simple technique involves carefully overlaying a sample of antiserum in a small glass tube with a solution of antigen so that a sharp interface is formed between the two layers. Diffusion between the two components occurs until an area of optimal concentrations develops. Where this occurs, a ring of precipitation is seen (fig. 13.2).

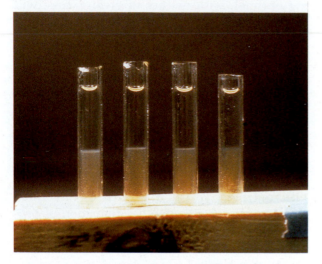

Figure 13.2   Ascoli Ring Test: the tubes show decreasing amounts of precipitate from left to right.

In order to perform this test, it is necessary to place the more dense antiserum in the bottom, and both solutions must be as clear as possible. Cloudiness in either solution may confuse the results. A normal serum control must always be used to detect nonspecific turbidity.

This technique is a useful qualitative tool for rapidly detecting the presence of an antigen/antibody reaction, and can be used to detect antibody produced by rabbits in response to protein antigen.

Materials for Part A:

- ☐ 6 pieces of glass tubing and tissue paper
- ☐ clay block and labeling tape
- ☐ 2 ml of rabbit antiserum against bovine serum albumin (rabbit anti-BSA)
- ☐ 0.5 ml of normal rabbit serum
- ☐ 1 ml of 1 % bovine serum albumin (BSA) in saline
- ☐ 4 test tubes

- ☐ 200 μl and 1000 μl automatic pipettes with tips
- ☐ 2 Pasteur pipettes and bulb

⚠ **Safety Tip:**
The glass tubing pieces may have sharp edges—handle with care.

Procedure:

1. Wipe the 6 pieces of tubing clean from fingerprints and dust with tissue. Stand the tubing pieces upright in the clay block.

2. Place a piece of tape on the block in front of the tubes for labeling (don't write on the tubes).

3. Using a Pasteur pipette, fill each of first 5 tubing pieces half full (no more) with antiserum; fill tube 6 half full with *normal* serum. Take care to place the tip of the Pasteur pipette all the way to the bottom of the tube so that the top will not become contaminated with antiserum. Avoid introducing air bubbles when adding the antiserum. *Never dilute the antiserum for this test.*

4. Prepare the following 10-fold dilutions of antigen in saline:

    1:10, 1:100, 1:1000, 1:10000.

    To do this, prepare 4 dilution blanks by adding 0.9 ml (900 μl) saline to each tube. Transfer 0.1 ml (100 μl) antigen solution through all tubes. Your instructor will demonstrate the proper use of the automatic pipettes.

5. Label the tape in front of the tubes with the appropriate antigen dilution. Label the fifth and sixth tubing pieces "antigen control," and "antiserum control."

6. Working back from the most dilute to the most concentrated, carefully layer each antigen dilution over the antiserum in the appropriate tube using one Pasteur pipette. Tube 5 is layered with saline alone, and tube 6 contains normal serum layered with the most concentrated antigen solution. To prevent mixing at the interface, hold the clay block at a slight slant and slowly introduce the antigen solution along the wall of the tube near the surface of the liquid.

7. After 10 minutes, examine the tubes for precipitation at the interface and record the results below. The reaction will disappear over time due to diffusion between the two layers.

Results of Ring Test for Detection of Anti-BSA Antibody
Result (+ or -)

BSA dilution				saline control	antiserum control
1:10	1:100	1:1000	1:10,000		

B. Ouchterlony Test (Double Gel Diffusion)

Because antisera are heterogeneous mixtures of antibodies and because there may be more than one antigen in even the purest preparations, multiple antigen/antibody reactions may be possible in a single mixture. Gel diffusion precipitation techniques allow the detection and examination of multiple reactions not possible with fluid medium.

The simplest gel diffusion technique was developed in 1946 by Oudin. This test involves incorporation of one of the reactants (usually antiserum) into agar contained in a test tube. The antigen solution is layered on top of the serum/ agarose mixture. The antigen solution will diffuse down into the agarose, and a line of visible precipitation will form at the equivalence zone for each antigen/antibody reaction (figure 13.3). In other words, each antigen will behave independently to combine with its homologous antibody. Once formed, the line of precipitation will not disperse.

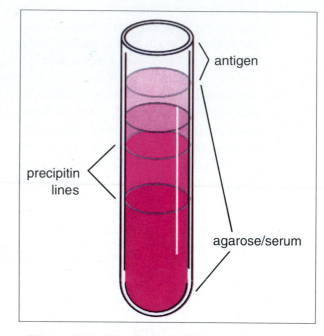

Figure 13.3   Simple Gel Diffusion Precipitation

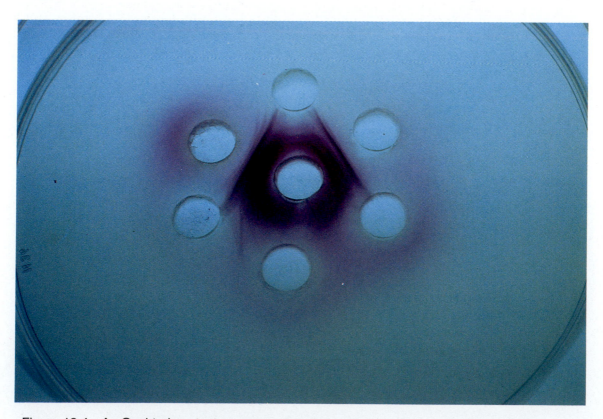

Figure 13.4   An Ouchterlony test on serum samples containing many proteins; lines of precipitation can be seen between the wells.

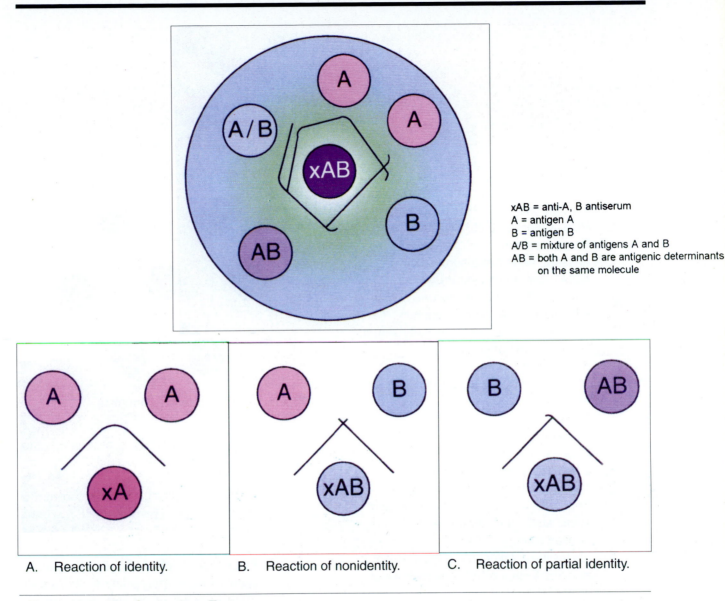

xAB = anti-A, B antiserum
A = antigen A
B = antigen B
A/B = mixture of antigens A and B
AB = both A and B are antigenic determinants
     on the same molecule

A. Reaction of identity.   B. Reaction of nonidentity.   C. Reaction of partial identity.

Figure 13.5 The Ouchterlony Test

The double diffusion technique developed by Organ Ouchterlony about 40 years ago adds an extra dimension to the simple tube diffusion method by utilizing diffusion of both reactants towards one another. A layer of melted agarose is poured into a petri plate. After solidification, small holes are cut in the agarose to form wells. These wells are filled with the appropriate antiserum and antigen reactants and incubated. Both reactants will diffuse toward one another, resulting in a narrow band of precipitation somewhere between the 2 wells where the equivalence zone is reached (fig. 13.4). Each band corresponds to a single antigen/antibody reaction. If several bands are evi-dent, there are at least that many antigen/antibody systems present. The relatedness of various antigens to one another as well as the relative concentrations of antigen and antibody can be elucidated by careful study of the pattern of bands and "spurs" appearing on the plate. (fig. 13.5).

For this exercise, you will perform 3 Ouchterlony tests to determine 1) the effect of dilution on placement of the equivalence zone, 2) the relationship of human serum components, and 3) the relationship of serum proteins between species.

Materials for Part B:
- ☐ 3 petri plates each containing 15 ml of 1% agarose + 2% PEG 6000 in
- ☐ PBS containing 0.05% NaN$_2$
- ☐ Pasteur pipette
- ☐ antisera: anti-bovine serum albumin (BSA), anti-human serum
- ☐ antigens: BSA, human serum, human IgG, human IgA, human albumin, porcine serum albumin, monkey serum, horse serum, rat serum
- ☐ 5 test tubes
- ☐ 200 μl and 1000 μl automatic pipettes and tips
- ☐ 5 mls saline
- ☐ staining dish
- ☐ PBS + 0.05% NaN$_2$
- ☐ 3 MM filter paper
- ☐ staining solution: 0.5% Coomassie Brilliant Blue R-250 dye in 10% glacial acetic acid, 40% ethanol, and 50% distilled water
- ☐ destaining solution: 5% glacial acetic acid, 15% ethanol, 80% distilled water

Procedure:

1. Label three plates A, B and C. Make sure to use a water-proof ink, and to label the bottom of the plates (agarose-containing side), but not in between wells where the precipitin lines will occur.

2. Place the plates over the template (fig. 13.6) to obtain the correct well pattern. Push the wide end of the Pasteur pipette into the agarose to punch the wells. Remove the agarose plugs from the wells by piercing them with the pipette tip, being careful not to distort the well

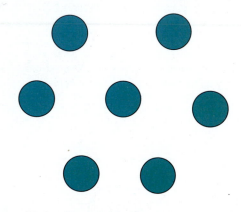

Figure 13.6   Ouchterlony Template

shape. Alternatively, a purchased template punch may be used.

3. Label the wells #1-#6 on the bottom of the plate (not in between wells), according to figure 13.7

4. Place 40–50 μl of the designated reagents in the appropriate wells as indicated for each of the tests (use only 15 μl if a template punch is used). Be *very* careful not to overfill the wells. Extra wells can be filled with saline as controls. To increase the amount of reagents at the precipitin lines, wells can be loaded 2 or 3 times (chased); allow all liquid to absorb into the agar before refilling with antigen.

5. Cover the plate (do not invert) and seal around the edges with tape to prevent drying. Incubate at room temp. for 48 hours.

6. Examine the precipitin lines for placement and presence of spurs. The plates

can be stained to see the lines more clearly, but be sure to record results before staining.

7. Place the petri plate in a staining dish containing PBS solution. Incubate at room temp. for 24 hours with gentle stirring to wash out unreacted proteins.

8. Remove the PBS and rinse the plate in water for 4 hours, then dry the agar by covering with filter paper and leaving overnight at room temp.

9. Submerge the agar plates in stain for 10 minutes at room temp. Decant the stain and rinse the plate in water. Destain in 2 to 3 changes of destaining solution or until the lines can be clearly resolved. Draw the results observed on figure 13.7.

Test A—effect of antigen dilution on the placement of the equivalence zone:

1. Place the anti-BSA in the center well.

2. Prepare the following serial 2-fold dilutions of BSA in saline; 1:2, 1:4, 1:8, 1:16, and 1:32. To do this, make 3 dilution blanks by placing 0.5 ml saline in each test tube. Transfer 0.5 ml BSA solution through all 5 tubes.

3. Fill the outer wells with undilute BSA solution and one of each of the prepared dilutions as shown in figure 13.7A.

Test B—The relationship of human serum components

1. Place anti-human serum in the center well.

2. Fill the outer wells with human serum, human serum albumin, human IgG, and human IgA as illustrated in figure 13.7B.

Test C—The evolutionary relationship of serum proteins

1. Fill the center well with anti-human serum.

2. Fill the outer wells with human serum, monkey serum, rat serum, pig serum, and horse serum as illustrated in figure 13.7C.

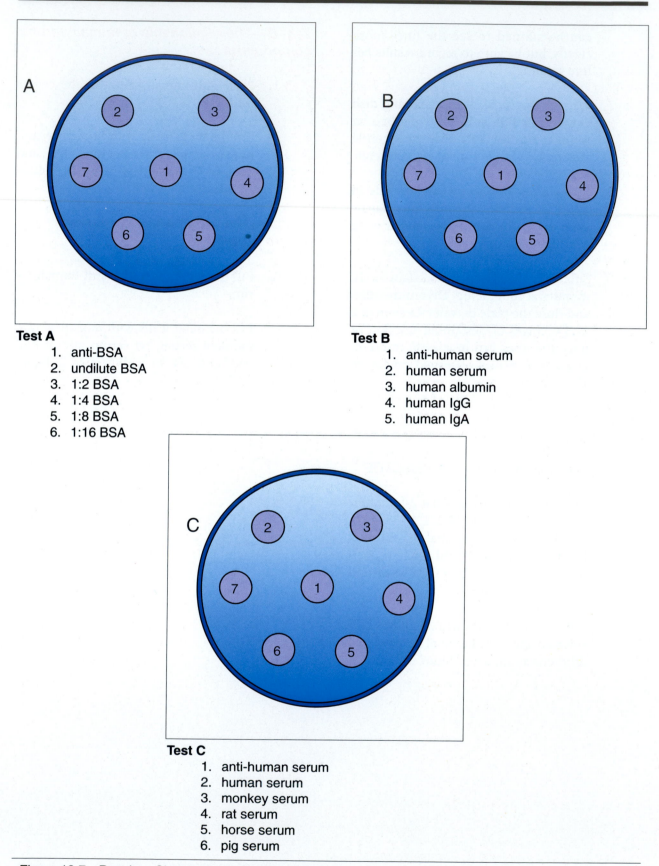

Test A
1. anti-BSA
2. undilute BSA
3. 1:2 BSA
4. 1:4 BSA
5. 1:8 BSA
6. 1:16 BSA

Test B
1. anti-human serum
2. human serum
3. human albumin
4. human IgG
5. human IgA

Test C
1. anti-human serum
2. human serum
3. monkey serum
4. rat serum
5. horse serum
6. pig serum

Figure 13.7 Results—Sketch above the precipitin lines which appeared on your plates.

C.   Mancini Test (Single Radial Diffusion)

Radial immunodiffusion is a variation of the simple agarose tube diffusion method of Oudin. Mancini extended the technique by incorporating the antiserum into a layer of agarose in a petri plate and placing the antigen in wells cut in the agarose. As the antigen diffuses outwards into the agarose, a ring of precipitation will develop around the well where the equivalence zone is reached (figure 13.8).

Mancini plates can be used to quantitate an unknown concentration of protein antigen. This is done by placing known concentrations of standard protein in the wells alongside the unknown. By plotting the square of the ring diameter versus protein concentration for each standard dilution, a standard curve can be constructed. The ring diameter of the unknown protein can then be fitted to the curve to determine its concentration (figure 13.9).

This technique is an important clinical method for monitoring serum protein level changes due to disease.

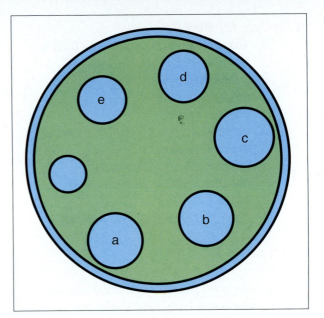

Figure 13.8   Mancini Test: Antigen solutions containing (a) 10 mg/ml, (b) 5 mg/ml, (c) 2.5 mg/ml, (d) 1.25 mg/ml, (e) 0.625 mg/ml protein incubated in a plate containing agarose gel with incorporated antiserum.

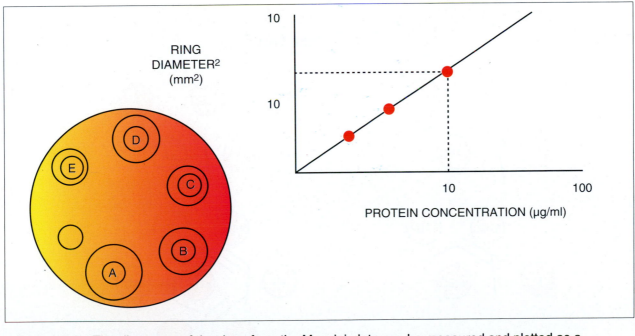

Figure 13.9   The diameters of the rings from the Mancini plate can be measured and plotted as a function of protein concentration.

Materials for Part C:

- ☐ 14 mls melted 1% agarose + 0.05% NaN_2 in PBS
- ☐ 1 ml antiserum
- ☐ empty petri plate
- ☐ Pasteur pipette
- ☐ sample of a protein antigen, 1% (10 mg/ml) in saline
- ☐ antigen solution of unknown concentration
- ☐ saline for dilutions
- ☐ 200 μl automatic pipette with tips

Procedure:

1. Remove the 14 mls melted agarose from the water bath. Add 1 ml antiserum, mix well, and quickly pour into the empty petri plate. Rock the plate to cover the surface evenly with agarose, then allow to solidify.

2. Place the plate over the template (use the one provided for the Ouchterlony test) and cut the outer ring of wells with the wide end of the Pasteur pipette. You do not need to cut out the center well. Remove the agarose from the wells being very careful not to gouge the agarose or distort the wells.

3. Prepare two-fold dilutions of the protein antigen in saline.

4. Label all wells with water-proof ink (on plate bottom) and fill each well with one of the standard dilutions or the unknown test sample.

5. Cover and seal the plate with tape (do not invert). Incubate at room temp. for 48 hours.

More Examples of Ouchterlony Tests:

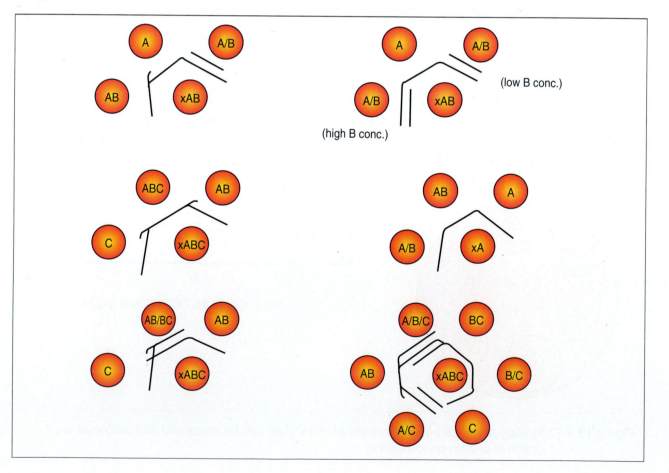

6. Measure the diameters of the rings with a ruler. Plot the standard curve below. Determine the concentration of the unknown sample from the curve. After measuring the rings, the plates can be washed, dried, and stained as for the Ouchterlony procedure.

Key Terms:

equivalence zone
double diffusion precipitation
radial immunodiffusion

Questions:

1. What is the main difference between the agglutination and precipitation reactions?

2. Why is the agglutination assay more sensitive than the precipitation assay?

3. In what situation would you expect to see more than one precipitin line between wells on an Ouchterlony plate?

Additional Reading:

1. Ouchterlony, O. 1949. Antigen-antibody reactions in gels. Acta Pathol. Microbiol. Scand. 26:507.

2. Oudin, J. 1952. Specific precipitation in gels and its application to immunochemical analysis. P. 335 *in* Methods in Medical Research, vol. 4, A. C. Corcoran, ed. Chicago, Illinois: Year Book Publishers.

3. Mancini, G., et al. 1965. Immunochemical quantitation of antigens by single radial immunodiffusion. Immunochemistry 2:235

4. Williams, C. A., and M. W. Chase, eds. 1971. Methods in Immunology and Immunochemistry, vol. 3. New York: Academic Press.

14 Immunoelectrophoresis

The main advantage of the Ouchterlony technique is the ability to resolve multiple antigen/antibody systems. However, this ability is limited because some mixtures are too complex to resolve. Immunoelectrophoresis (IEP) overcomes this problem by combining double gel diffusion with electrophoresis.

Electrophoresis is the movement of charged molecules through an electric field. Most proteins are charged molecules and will exhibit electrophoretic migration dependent on the pH of the buffer through which the proteins travel. In acid solutions, the amino groups of proteins are positively charged while the carboxyl groups are not charged. In a basic or alkaline solution, the carboxyl groups are negatively charged while the amino groups are not charged. Therefore, in the alkaline buffers commonly used for electrophoresis, most proteins have a net negative charge and will migrate toward the **anode** (+ electrode). At the same time, the buffer components assume a positive charge and move toward the **cathode** (− electrode) in a process known as **electroosmosis**. Some proteins, such as gamma globulin, are too weakly charged to overcome the electroosmotic forces and will actually be "back-washed" toward the cathode.

In immunoelectrophoresis, the protein sample to be examined is first separated into its components by electrophoresis through an agarose gel. The gel layer is prepared on a glass slide and the sample is placed in a well cut in the gel (figure 14.1). The slide is then placed in an electric field. Because each protein will have a characteristic net charge at a given pH, the proteins will migrate different distances in the gel. When the electrophoretic separation is completed, the proteins are resolved by double diffusion with antiserum. The antiserum is placed in a long trough cut into the gel parallel to the direction of protein migration.

The antiserum and the proteins, from their positions in the gel, will diffuse toward one another to form arcs of precipitation (fig. 14.2). This technique allows resolution of multiple components with similar electrophoretic mobilities by their antigenic differences, and at the same time resolves antigenically related components by their electrophoretic properties.

The blood, as you have seen, contains many components, including cellular elements (RBCs, WBCs, and platelets), as well as a variety of small molecules and proteins. The serum proteins consist of antibodies and many others which function as hormones or carrier molecules for the transport of metals, fatty acids, or amino acids.

The IEP technique has been used to identify the many proteins found in serum, and is often utilized in the diagnosis of serum protein disorders such as agammaglobulinemia or myelomas.

For this exercise you will analyze the components of your own serum.

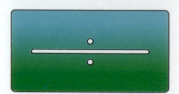

(a) Cut agarose and place antigen sample in well

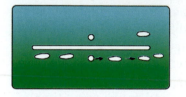

(b) Electrophorese the antigen sample

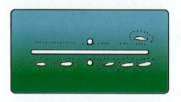

(c) Add antiserum to trough and incubate 48 hours

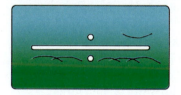

(d) Observe arcs of precipitation

Figure 14.1   Immunoelectrophoresis procedure

A.   Preparation of Agarose Slides

Materials for Part A:
☐ small bottle of 70% ethanol
☐ electrophoresis slides and frames
☐ melted adhesive agar (2% agarose in barbital buffer), held at 45°C

☐ melted immunoelectrophoresis agar (1% agarose in barbital buffer), held at 45°C
☐ held at 45°C
☐ small paint brush
☐ 10-ml pipette
☐ humid chamber
☐ refrigerator

Procedure:

1. Clean the glass slides with ethanol and wipe dry with tissue.

2. Load the electrophoresis frame with six glass slides, leaving about 2 cm between the ends of the outer slides and the edge of the frame. Make sure the slides remain tightly together.

3. "Paint" a thin layer of adhesive agar on the glass slides using a small paint brush and allow to set for 15 minutes. The adhesive agar allows adherence of the electrophoresis agar to the glass slide and ensures that the serum samples do not run out of the wells between the glass and the gel layer.

4. Heat a 10-ml pipette by sucking up the melted electrophoresis agar several times. Fill the small spaces at each end of the frame, then fill the frame so that each half contains 12 mls of the melted agar in a uniform layer. Allow to set for 15 minutes.

5. Place the slides in a humid chamber at 4°C until the next lab period.

⚠ **Safety Tips:**
1.   **Do not exchange lancets.**
2.   **Handle only your own serum.**
3.   **Dispose of lancets, cotton balls, bandages, and the like only in the container provided for that purpose.**

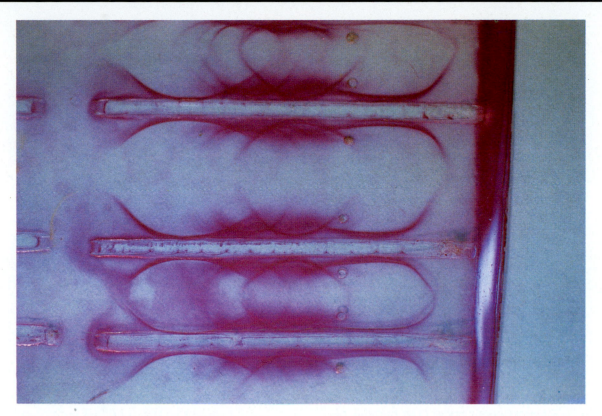

Figure 14.2   Immunoelectrophoresis of human serum samples with rabbit anti-human antiserum.

B.   Preparation of Human Serum Sample

Materials for Part B:
- ☐ 70% ethanol or alcohol swab
- ☐ sterile lancet
- ☐ cotton ball and bandage
- ☐ small glass tube or Eppendorf tube
- ☐ 2 Eppendorf tubes
- ☐ Pasteur pipette and bulb

Procedure:

1. Have a sterile lancet and a clean, dry cotton ball ready. Clean your left "ring" finger tip with an alcohol-soaked cotton ball and let it air dry.

2. Puncture your finger with the lancet, trying to strike at the side of the finger tip to avoid the calloused skin in the center. Discard the first drop of blood by wiping it away with the cotton ball.

3. Allow 5 drops of blood to collect in a small tube.

4. Label the tube with your name and let the blood clot on the bench for 20 to 30 minutes.

> ⚠ *Safety Tips:*
> 1.   The electrophoresis buffer contains barbital, a poison. Wear safety gloves at all times during this part of the procedure.
> 2.   Never open the lid or place hands inside the electrophoresis chamber while in use.
> 3.   Never remove or insert the electrical leads unless the power supply is turned off. Start with the power off and the voltage and current turned all the way down to zero before connecting the leads (red to red and black to black), then turn on and bring voltage and current up slowly to desired level. Reverse this procedure to disconnect the gel. If a gel is disconnected before turning off the power, considerable electrical energy remains in the power unit and can discharge through the sockets even though the unit is turned off.
> 4.   Always remove leads one at a time with the other hand free or on a nonconducting surface. Using both hands can create a very dangerous shunt of current across the chest and through the heart if you contact a bare wire.

C.   Sample Electrophoresis

Materials for Part C:
☐ Electrophoresis buffer (Tris-barbital, pH 8.8)
☐ gel punch and vacuum apparatus
☐ 1 µl human serum sample
☐ 1 µl human serum albumin/bromophenol blue dye sample
☐ electrophoresis apparatus with power supply
☐ 20 µl automatic pipette with tips
☐ 4 microporous wicks

Procedure:

1.   Cut the immunoelectrophoresis pattern (wells and trough) in the agar over each glass slide using the cutting device provided. Remove the agar from the two wells *only* (not the trough). Be careful not to damage the walls of the wells.

2.   Carefully deposit 1 µl of serum in one well, and 1 ml of the albumin/bromophenol blue mixture in the opposite well (do not overfill wells).

3.   Place the frame in the electrophoresis apparatus so that it bridges both chambers.

4.   Fill the chambers with electrophoresis buffer. Wet four wicks per frame in the buffer, and place one end of each on the agar surface and let the other end hang into the buffer.

5.   Connect the power source, using the red lead for the anode (+) and the black lead for the cathode (−). Run for 120 minutes at about 3 to 5 milliamps per frame (150 Volts), or until the bromophenol dye reaches the + electrode end of the gel. Check the movement of the dye shortly after starting the run. It should be moving toward the anode.

6.   After electrophoresis, turn off all power to the unit and disconnect the leads. Remove the frames from the apparatus.

D. Double Diffusion

Materials for Part D:
- ☐ gel knife
- ☐ 20 µl anti-human serum (rabbit)
- ☐ 20 µl automatic pipette and tips
- ☐ humid chamber
- ☐ refrigerator
- ☐ 37°C incubator

Procedure:

1. Cut across each end of the trough with the gel knife and remove the agar.

2. Place about 100 µl of antiserum into the trough (do not overfill) with an automatic pipette and spread evenly in the trough.

3. Incubate the slides in a humid chamber at 4°C for 2 days.

E. Staining

Materials for Part E:
- ☐ staining dish (polystyrene or glass)
- ☐ 0.3 M NaCl
- ☐ 0.15 M NaCl
- ☐ staining solution: acid fuchsin, 0.2% in methanol, acetic acid, and distilled H_2O (5:1:4)
- ☐ destaining solution: methanol/acetic acid/distilled H_2O (5:1:4)

⚠ Safety Tip:
Wear gloves to avoid contact with staining and destaining solutions. These solutions can damage clothing.

Procedure:

1. Wash the slides 24 to 48 hours in 2 changes of cold 0.3 M NaCl and 2 changes of 0.15 M NaCl, to rinse remaining unreacted serum and antiserum out of the gel matrix.

2. Fill the trough with distilled water and cover the agar with a piece of filter paper cut to the size of the slide. Make sure there are no bubbles in the trough. Saturate the filter paper with water and incubate at 37°C until completely dry.

3. Place the slides in the staining dish and cover with staining solution for 10 minutes.

4. Decant the stain and submerge the slides in destaining solution for about 15–20 minutes, with 2–3 changes of destaining solution.

5. Remove the slides and air dry. The slides may now be kept indefinitely. Examine the slide and identify the arcs of precipitation below. Draw the precipitation pattern on figure 14.3 below.

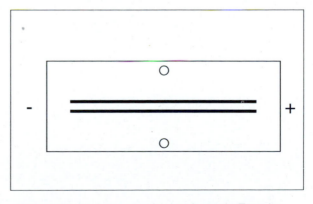

Figure 14.3   Immunoelectrophoresis Results

Key Terms:

electrophoresis
electroosmosis
anode
cathode

Questions:

1. What is the purpose of the bromo-phenol blue dye added to the albumin sample?

2. What results might you observe on immunoelectrophoresis of the serum from patients with a) agammaglobulinemia, b) multiple myeloma?

Additional Reading:

1. Williams, C. A. 1960. Immunoelectro-phoresis. Sci. Am. 110:130.

2. Jeppsson, J. O., et al. 1979. Agarose gel electrophoresis. Clin. Chem. 25:629

3. Doolittle, R. F. 1985. Proteins. Sci. Am. 253(4):88

4. Tonegawa, S. 1985. The molecules of the immune system. Sci. Am. 253(4):122.

15 The Quantitative Precipitin Assay

In Exercise 13 you carried out several types of qualitative assays that utilize the precipitation reaction. Qualitative assays have many applications in the identification of various antigens and the detection of antibody. In this exercise you will carry out the *quantitative* precipitin assay. This assay is a highly accurate method for deriving unknown antigen concentrations and may also be used to illustrate the characteristics of the precipitation reaction.

As you learned in exercise 13, antibody reacts with soluble antigens to form a "lattice structure," or visible precipitate. If you mix a fixed quantity of antibody with increasing concentrations of antigen, it can be seen that the amount of precipitate formed starts out small, increases to a maximum quantity, then decreases again. By plotting the amount of precipitate formed versus the antigen concentration used, a precipitin curve can be generated (fig. 15.1). Little precipitate is formed when the antibody is in great excess and all antigenic sites are saturated (the prozone), or when antigen is in great excess and all antibody binding sites are saturated (the postzone; see also fig. 13.1). The greatest amount of precipitate is formed at some optimal concentration near the equivalence zone, usually at a very slight antibody excess. The equivalence zone is the point when neither antibody nor antigen can be found unbound in the supernatant fluid.

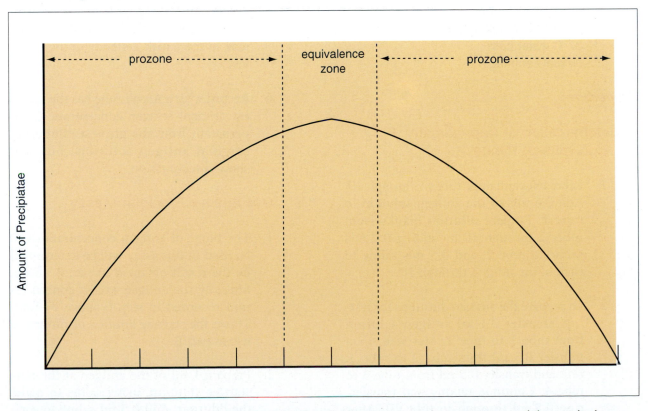

Figure 15.1   A precipitin curve, showing zones of antibody excess, antigen excess, and the equivalence zone.

For this exercise, you will generate a precipitin curve by mixing varying amounts of antigen with a constant amount of antibody. You will begin by determining a good concentration of antibody to use in the assay. Then you will carry out the precipitin assay and collect the precipitate and the supernatant from each tube. The Bio-Rad assay will be used to determine the amount of precipitate formed at each antigen dilution, and the Ascoli ring test will be used to observe how much antigen or antibody remains in the supernatant after each precipitate forms. You should review exercises 7 and 13 for the Bio-Rad assay and Ascoli ring test procedures.

Materials:

- ☐ antigen: Bovine serum albumin (BSA), 0.1% in saline
- ☐ antiserum: anti-BSA, diluted 1:2 in saline
- ☐ 16 15-ml centrifuge tubes
- ☐ 20 mls normal saline
- ☐ clay block
- ☐ 10 Ascoli ring tubes
- ☐ 40 small test tubes
- ☐ 100 mls Bio-Rad reagent
- ☐ 37°C water bath
- ☐ clinical centrifuge

Procedure:

A. Determination of Approximate Equivalence Range

1. Label ten centrifuge tubes 1 through 10. Add 0.6 mls of the antigen solution to tube 1. Prepare dilution blanks from tubes 2 through 10 by adding 0.9 mls saline to tube 2, and 0.5 mls saline to each of the tubes 3 through 10.

2. To prepare the antigen dilutions for testing, transfer 0.1 ml antigen solution from tube 1 to tube 2. Mix well, then transfer 0.5 ml from tube 2 to tube 3. Mix and transfer 0.5 ml from tube 3 to tube 4. Continue mixing and transferring 0.5 ml through to tube 10. After mixing, discard 0.5 ml from tube 10. You now have the original antigen solu-

tion in tube 1, a 1:10 dilution of the original antigen solution in tube 2, and 1:2 dilutions ranging from 1:20 in tube 3 to 1:2560 in tube 10.

3. Add 0.5 mls of antibody to each tube and mix the tubes. Place the tubes in a 37°C water bath for 30 minutes.

4. Centrifuge the tubes at $2,500 \times g$ for 10 minutes. Meanwhile, place ten Ascoli ring tubes in a clay block and fill each halfway full with anti-BSA antiserum.

5. When centrifugation is complete, carefully overlay the supernatant from each of the tubes 1 through 10 onto the anti-BSA in the Ascoli tubes. Incubate the Ascoli tubes for 15 minutes at room temperature, then look for tubes which have a ring of precipitate at the interface. The tube or tubes showing precipitate represent the zone of antigen excess. That is, excess antigen was left in the supernatant after the first incubation (step 3), and was able to react with antibody in the Ascoli test.

6. Record which Ascoli tube has the smallest original antigen concentration (supernatant from the greatest dilution of original antigen solution) but still shows precipitation.

B. Quantitative Precipitin Assay

1. The range of antigen concentrations to be used in this assay will be determined by the result obtained in part A above. Multiply the antigen excess concentration recorded in step 6 above by four. This is the starting dilution of antigen to use in part B.

2. Prepare 1 ml of the antigen at the new starting dilution, using saline to make the dilution. Add 0.5 ml saline to each of six centrifuge tubes. Prepare two-fold dilutions from the new starting dilution

through the six saline tubes for a total of seven tubes. Discard 0.5 mls from the last dilution (7th tube). These dilutions should span the equivalence zone.

3. Add 0.5 mls of anti-BSA to each of the seven tubes. Mix the tubes and incubate in a 37°C water bath for 30 minutes.

4. Mix the tubes very gently, then place in a refrigerator until the next lab period.

Next lab period

5. After refrigeration centrifuge the tubes at 2,500 × g for 10 minutes. Carefully decant the supernatant from each tube into a separate test tube and save both the supernatants and the pellets. Be careful not to lose any of the precipitate pellet.

6. Place two rows of seven small test tubes in a rack (14 tubes total). Label these tubes 1A–7A and 1B–7B. Add 0.3 mls of 0.1% BSA to each of 1A–7A, and 0.3 mls of anti-BSA to each of 1B–7B. Add 0.3 mls of each of the supernatants saved from the previous step to the corresponding tube of BSA (row A) and a tube of anti-BSA (row B).

7. Incubate the 14 tubes for 30 minutes in a 37°C water bath, then look for precipitate. Precipitate should form in the last few tubes of row A. This is the zone of antibody excess. Precipitate should also form in the first few tubes of row B. This is the zone of antigen excess.

8. To determine the amount of precipitate formed in each pellet, conduct the Bio-Rad assay for protein determination. Dissolve each precipitate pellet in 1 ml of saline. Prepare a standard curve from BSA

as described in exercise 7, then determine the concentration of each precipitate by adding 0.1 ml of each dissolved precipitate to 5 mls of Bio-Rad reagent and reading spectrophotometrically.

9. Make a graph of the antigen concentrations versus amount of precipitate formed, and designate which area of the curve represents antigen excess and which area represents antibody excess.

Questions:

1. Explain what is meant by the terms "prozone," "postzone," and "equivalence zone" in precipitation reactions.

2. How would you design a procedure using the quantitative precipitin assay to measure the amounts of a particular bacterial toxin present in spoiled foods?

Additional Reading:

1. Kabat, E. A., and M. M. Mayer. 1961. Experimental Immunochemistry. Springfield, Illinois: Charles C. Thomas.

2. Martin, D. S. 1943. A simplified serum dilution method for quantitative titration of precipitin in a pure antigen-antibody system. J. Lab. Clin. Med. 28:1477.

3. Garvey, J. S., et al. 1977. Methods in Immunology. A Laboratory Text for Instruction and Research. Reading, Massachusetts: Benjamin/Cummings. Pgs. 347–374.

4. Haber, E., and R. M. Krause, eds. 1977. Antibodies in Human Diagnosis and Therapy. New York: Raven Press.

16 Complement Fixation Assay

Complement is the collective term for a system of serum proteins found in warm-blooded animals. These proteins were discovered in 1894 by Pfeiffer, who noticed that the bacterium Vibrio cholerae was lysed by some factor present in immune serum. The factor was originally called **Alexin** ("to ward off"), but was later renamed **complement** ("to make complete") by Paul Ehrlich.

Complement consists of at least 20 proteins and glycoproteins which carry out enzymatic reactions in a sequential, or "cascade" fashion. The proteins are extremely labile, being inactivated merely by shaking, prolonged storage, or heating to 56°C for 30 minutes.

Complement mediates a variety of biological reactions such as opsonization, increased capillary permeability, chemotaxis, and lysis of cells. Although these functions are all important in the process of *inflammation*, complement is not a product of an immune response but is present at all times in normal serum. For this reason, complement can be considered a "nonspecific" barrier to infection.

Two properties allow complement to be useful for the detection of antigen or antibody in the complement fixation test; the nonspecific binding of complement to antigen-antibody complexes, and the ability to lyse antibody-sensitized cells. In this test (fig. 16.1), antigen and a serum sample, which may or may not contain the homologous antibody, are mixed and incubated with complement. If antibody specific for the antigen is present in the serum, antigen-antibody complexes will form and some or all of the available complement will be bound by the complexes (fixed). However, if the suspected antibody is not present, the complement will not be fixed but will be left unbound and free in solution. Because the binding of complement by an antigen-antibody complex cannot be seen, a visual indicator system is necessary. The indicator is a mixture of sheep erythrocytes and rabbit anti-sheep erythrocyte antiserum (hemolysin), and really functions as a secondary antigen-antibody complex of sensitized cells. If any complement is left unfixed in the first step, subsequent addition of the indicator in the second step will result in the fixation of complement by the sensitized erythrocytes followed by lysis of the cells (a negative reaction). If an antigen-antibody reaction had occurred in the first step, thus fixing all the available complement, the indicator cells would *not* lyse (a positive reaction).

The complement fixation assay offers a distinct advantage in that either soluble or particulate antigens may be employed. The assay is an even more sensitive serological procedure than precipitation or agglutination, but requires careful preliminary standardization of the reagents. Standardization procedures (part A) will be carried out by your instructor. You will perform the test proper (part B), using the appropriate controls.

A. Standardization of Reagents

Standardization of the test reagents involves titration of each to determine the concentrations and conditions optimal for the most sensitive measurement of complement fixation. All procedures are carried out in veronal buffered saline containing $MgSO_4$ and $CaCl_2$. These ions are necessary for the stability and function of complement.

The standardization procedures include:

1. Titration to determine the antigen dilution which will detect a small amount of antibody by complement fixation.

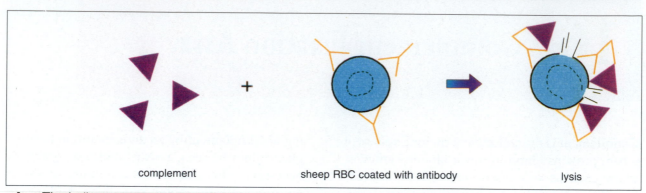

A. The indicator system (sheep RBCs coated with antibody to sheep RCBs) is lysed in the presence of complement.

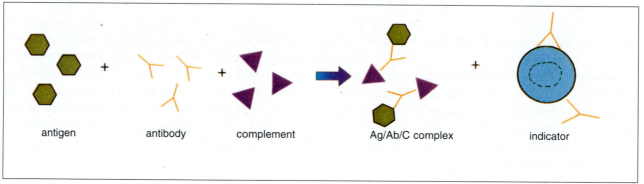

B. A positive test: if another Antigen/Antibody system is present, complement will no longer be available to lyse the indicator.

Figure 16.1   The Complement Fixation Test.

2. Titration of the correct amount of hemolysin which will bind to erythrocytes to give maximum hemolysis.

3. Titration of the amount of complement which will give 50% hemolysis (one CH_{50} unit), a range in which the lysis of sensitized erythrocytes is most sensitive to small changes in complement concentration.

B. Complement Fixation Assay

Materials:

- ☐ 5 mls veronal-buffered saline (VBS) with $MgSO_4$ and $CaCl_2$
- ☐ 6 mls hemolysin (standardized to contain 2 units/ml)
- ☐ 6 mls sheep erythrocytes (standardized to 2% in VBS)
- ☐ 5 mls guinea pig complement (standardized to contain 5 units/ml in VBS)
- ☐ 5 mls antigen (standardized in VBS)
- ☐ 1.5 mls antiserum (inactivated for 30 minutes at 56°C)
- ☐ 11 test tubes
- ☐ 1000 µl automatic pipette and tips
- ☐ 6 10-ml pipettes
- ☐ 37°C water bath

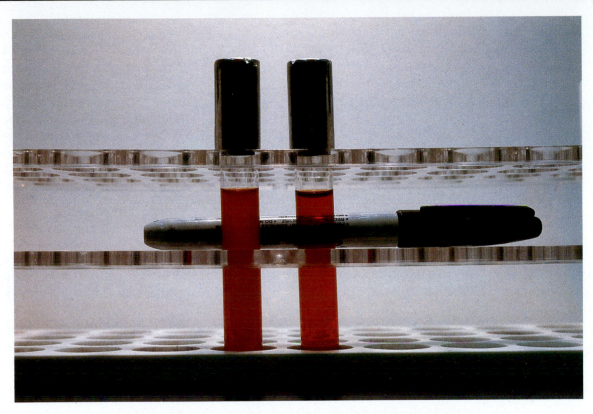

Figure 16.2   Positive (turbid) and negative (lysis) complement fixation tests.

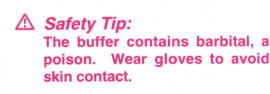

⚠ *Safety Tip:*
The buffer contains barbital, a poison. Wear gloves to avoid skin contact.

Procedure:

The complement is kept at 4°C. Do not remove it until just before use!

1. Label 10 empty tubes 1 through 10. Tubes 1 through 6 will compose the test, tubes 7 through 10 will be controls (see table 16.1).

2. With a 10-ml pipette, add VBS to tubes 7 through 10 as indicated in table 16.1. The VBS is used to equalize volumes in all tubes.

3. With an automatic pipette, add 0.5 ml (500 µl) of antiserum to tubes 1 and 8.

4. Prepare serial 2-fold dilutions of the antiserum in tube 1 through tube 6. To do this, transfer 500 µl from tube 1 to tube 2, mix, then with a new tip transfer 500 µl from tube 2 to tube 3. Continue transferring 500 µl through to tube 6, using a new pipette tip for each transfer. Discard 500 µl from tube 6 when finished.

5. Using a 10-ml pipette, add 0.5 ml antigen solution to all tubes except 8, 9, and 10

6. Using a 10-ml pipette, add 0.5 ml complement to all tubes except 10.

7. Mix the tubes by *gently* shaking the rack (do not vortex—remember complement is labile), then place the tubes in a 37°C water bath for 30 minutes. While the tubes are incubating, prepare the sensitized erythrocyte indicator by mix-

ing the 6 mls of 2% erythrocytes with the 6 mls of hemolysin in one tube.

8. After the 30 minute incubation, add 1 ml of sensitized erythrocytes to all tubes.

9. Mix the tubes by gently shaking the rack and return to the 37°C water bath. Incubate again for 30 minutes.

10. Observe your control tubes. Tubes which are – (no complement fixed) are clear due to hemolysis. Tubes which are + (complement was fixed) are turbid due to unlysed erythrocytes. Tube 7 tests for anticomplementary factors in the antigen preparation that could affect the complement and prevent it from lysing the erythrocytes. It should be completely hemolysed. Tube 8 tests for

anticomplementary factors in the antiserum and should also be hemolysed. Tube 9 tests whether the amount of complement added is correct and sufficient to lyse the sensitized erythrocytes. It should hemolyze completely. Tube 10 demonstrates that the sensitized erythrocytes will not lyse on their own in saline without complement present. It should not show hemolysis.

11. If the control tubes show the expected results, read tubes 1 through 6. The titer of the antiserum is expressed as the reciprocal of the last (most dilute) tube which still contains enough antibody to inhibit hemolysis. In other words, the endpoint is the last dilution showing any degree of turbidity, with the next tube exhibiting complete hemolysis. Record your results in table 16.1.

Table 16.1   Procedure for Complement Fixation Test

Tube no.	mls antigen	mls serum	mls Compl.	mls VBS	mls indicator	result
1	0.5	0.5	0.5	–	1	
2	0.5		0.5	–	1	
3	0.5		0.5	–	1	
4	0.5		0.5	–	1	
5	0.5		0.5	–	1	
6	0.5		0.5	–	1	
7	0.5	–	0.5	0.5	1	(–)
8	–	0.5	0.5	0.5	1	(–)
9	–	–	0.5	1.0	1	(–)
10	–	–	–	1.5	1	(+)

Key Terms:

complement
chemotaxis
hemolysin
indicator
hemolysis

Questions:

1. Why is the serum used in this test heated to 56°C prior to use?

2. Describe how each control works in the complement fixation test.

3. What kinds of antigens can be used in the complement fixation test?

Additional Reading:

1. Osler, A. S. 1961. Functions of the complement system. Adv. Immunol. 132–210.

2. Muller-Eberhard, H. J. 1975. Complement. Ann. Rev. Biochem. 44:697.

3. Rother, K., and G. O. Till, eds. 1988. The Complement System. New York: Springer-Verlag.

4. Lambris, J. D. 1988. The multifunctional role of C3, the third component of complement. Immunol. Today 9(12):387.

17   Western Blot

Immunoelectrophoresis is one method used to resolve different protein antigens in a complex mixture. Another procedure which is rapidly replacing more conventional methods of identifying mixed proteins is a technique called the **Western blot** or **Immunoblot**. This technique is used extensively in research laboratories for the determination of antigen characteristics, the detection of antigens that are difficult to label or precipitate, the purification of antibodies, and assay of the presence, quantity, and specificity of antibodies from different sera. The technique is also useful in clinical diagnosis for detection of specific antibody in serum or proteins of disease agents in clinical specimens. The most notable example is the detection of the AIDS virus. Any of the viral structural proteins can be found in a clinical sample by a Western blot analysis.

The procedure can be broken down into three stages (figure 17.1). Stage one involves gel electrophoresis of the protein mixture to resolve each component as a separate band (similar to the immunoelectrophoresis technique). In the second stage, the proteins are transferred from their positions in the gel to a nitrocellulose membrane. This is called "blotting." The third stage involves "staining" the membrane to visualize the transferred proteins so that they can be identified both by their electrophoretic migration pattern and their antigenic characteristics. The staining may be done either as a direct method, or more commonly, as an indirect method.

In the direct method, the antigens are detected by incubating the membrane in a solution of specific antibody. Because an antigen/antibody complex can't be seen on the membrane, the antibody must be labeled with some type of visual marker or "tag." The tag in turn must be a molecule which can bind to an antibody molecule without destroying the antibody's specific binding ability.

Chromogenic enzymes (enzymes which bring about a color change in a colorless substrate), radioactive isotopes, or fluorescent dyes have all been utilized as antibody tags for various labeling procedures, but enzymes and radioisotopes are usually used for the Western blot.

In the indirect method, the membrane is first incubated in a solution of unlabeled primary antibody. The primary antibody, if bound to an antigen on the membrane, can then be detected by incubating the membrane in a solution of labeled secondary antibody which is specific for the immunoglobulin class of the primary antibody (produced by immunizing an animal from a different species with the primary antibody). Gelatin is added to the membrane during antibody incubation to minimize non-specific protein binding. This is called "blocking." Proteins other than gelatin may also be used as long as they are unrelated to the antigens used in the assay.

The indirect method can be used both to identify unknown antigens using primary antibody of known specificity, or to detect specific antibody in serum using a known antigen. This method has several other advantages over the direct method. First, because the primary antibody itself has several antigenic epitopes, several secondary antibody molecules could bind to each primary antibody molecule. Thus, if the secondary antibody is labeled, then for every antigen several labeled molecules will be bound rather than only one. This has the obvious effect of amplifying the label, thereby making the test more sensitive. Secondly, it is more efficient to prepare only one, species-specific, labeled secondary antibody than different labeled primary antibodies for every possible antigen being tested.

In this exercise, you will examine serum proteins by performing a Western blot.

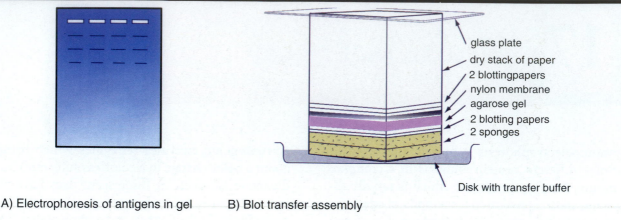

A) Electrophoresis of antigens in gel   B) Blot transfer assembly

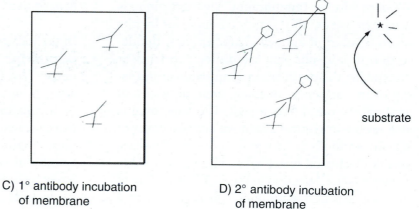

glass plate
dry stack of paper
2 blottingpapers
nylon membrane
agarose gel
2 blotting papers
2 sponges

Disk with transfer buffer

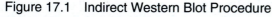
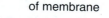

C) 1° antibody incubation
of membrane

D) 2° antibody incubation
of membrane

substrate

Figure 17.1   Indirect Western Blot Procedure

A.   Preparing the Gel

Several different types of support materials can be used for the electrophoresis of proteins. These include cellulose acetate paper, starch blocks, and agar, agarose, or polyacrylamide gels. Polyacrylamide is the material of choice for clear resolution of proteins. However, the use of a polyacrylamide gel for the Western blot requires an electrophoretic transfer device. Furthermore, acrylamide gels are fairly fragile and are composed of toxic reagents. You will use a polyacrylamide gel in exercise 28 in a procedure that does not require as much handling of the gel. In this exercise you will see how agarose can also be used to separate proteins for the Western blot.

To separate proteins on an agarose gel, a fairly tight gel matrix is required. This can be achieved by using 7% agarose instead of the 1% agarose usually used for larger nucleic acid molecules. A 7% gel made from regular agarose is extremely viscous and difficult to pour into a gel casting plate. However, special formulations of agarose have been designed which allow preparation of high percentage gels.

Materials for Part A:

- ☐ gel casting tray and comb
- ☐ NuSieve™ GTG agarose
- ☐ gel buffer (Tris-borate, pH 8.6)
- ☐ large flask
- ☐ boiling water bath
- ☐ 48°C water bath
- ☐ Pasteur pipette and bulb
- ☐ plastic wrap

Procedure:

1. Assemble the gel casting tray on a level work surface.

2. Prepare a suspension of NuSieve (10.5 grams/150 mls) in gel buffer in a flask. Melt the agarose by placing the flask in a boiling water bath until the solution becomes clear and viscous. There should

be no more "grains" of agarose left. After melting completely, gently swirl the agarose to mix completely, then place the agarose in a 48°C water bath for 15 minutes or until you are able to comfortably hold the flask in your hand. During this time, do not shake the agarose again because it would introduce air bubbles in the gel.

3. Using a Pasteur pipette, seal any edges or cracks that are present in the gel casting tray with a little of the melted agarose. Allow this to cool and harden.

4. Carefully pour the remainder of the agarose into the tray. Immediately place the well-forming comb into position in the casting tray at the cathode (black) end of the gel.

5. After the gel has cooled (at least 20 minutes at room temperature or 10 to 15 minutes in a refrigerator), carefully remove the comb, as well as the end pieces of the casting tray if present. If the gel is to be stored for later use, leave the end pieces and comb in place and wrap the tray in plastic wrap. Store the gel in the refrigerator.

B. Sample Preparation

Electrophoretic separation of proteins by molecular size requires SDS treatment and denaturation of the proteins. Sodium dodecyl sulfate (SDS) is an anionic detergent which binds to the protein and masks its charge with its own negative charge. The protein is also denatured with β-mercaptoethanol (a reducing agent) which cleaves disulfide bonds and causes the polypeptide chains to dissociate and unfold. Thus treated, the proteins assume a rod-like shape and all carry the same net negative charge. The only characteristic property left to each protein is its particular molecular size. The proteins can now be separated by their ability to make their way through the small pores of the gel matrix.

Materials for Part B:

- [ ] whole human serum and samples of individual human serum proteins
- [ ] 2X SDS sample buffer
- [ ] protein molecular weight standards in sample buffer (high range)
- [ ] Eppendorf tubes
- [ ] heat-resistant rack
- [ ] boiling water bath
- [ ] straight pins
- [ ] 20 µl automatic pipette with tips
- [ ] agarose gel in electrophoresis unit
- [ ] TBE/SDS electrophoresis buffer

> ⚠ **Safety Tips:**
> If obtaining a sample of your own serum, follow the procedure and safety tips given in exercise 14, part B. If you are being given a human serum sample to use, treat it as potentially infectious, and wear gloves during use.

Procedure:

1. If using your own serum, obtain a small serum sample by the methods outlined in exercise 14, part B. Mix 10 µl of serum and 10 µl of each serum protein with equal volumes of 2X sample buffer in Eppendorf tubes. Also mix the standard protein mixture with an equal volume of 2X sample buffer if not already done. Tap the tubes lightly with your finger to mix the contents.

2. Pierce the tops of the tubes with a pin to vent steam. Place the serum and protein sample and molecular weight standard tubes in a heat-resistant floating rack.

3. Being careful not to submerge the tubes in water, place the rack in vigorously boiling water for 5 minutes. Meanwhile, place the agarose gel in the electrophoresis chamber, making sure the wells are at the cathode end of the chamber.

Slowly fill the chamber with enough electrophoresis buffer to just cover the gel by 2 or 3 mm.

4. Using the automatic pipette and a new tip for each sample, place 10 µl of each sample into a well in the gel. This is most easily done by placing your pipetting arm with the elbow resting on the lab bench, and supporting the arm with your other hand to steady it. Place the pipette tip just above the well before slowly ejecting the sample. Do not place the tip into the well as you might move the gel or jab through the bottom of the well. The glycerol in the sample will cause it to sink and remain at the bottom of the well.

C.   Electrophoresis

The buffer used for electrophoresis contains SDS to maintain the proteins in their negatively charged state. The buffer also has a moderately high ionic strength to permit rapid protein migration resulting in sharper protein migration zones. Very high ionic strength buffers can cause too much heat production during electrophoresis, which leads to distortion of the protein bands. Some electrophoresis units are equipped with sophisticated cooling mechanisms to help overcome this problem. The electrophoresis is conducted with a constant voltage of 150 V and variable amperage.

Materials for Part C:
☐ gel and electrophoresis unit
☐ power supply and cables

Procedure:

1. Cover the electrophoresis chamber with the lid.

2. With the power supply off, connect the cables from the power supply to the unit; black to black (–) and red to red (+) (fig. 17.2).

3. Turn on the power and raise the voltage slowly to 150 volts. Check the unit to make sure the cables are connected properly. There should be small bubbles rising from the platinum wires of the unit, and the samples should begin to move toward the anode. Electrophorese until the bromophenol blue in the samples has migrated at least 4 inches.

4. When the run is completed, turn the voltage down to zero, turn off the power supply, and disconnect the cables.

⚠ **Safety Tips:**
1. **Never open the lid or place hands inside the electrophoresis chamber while in use.**
2. **Never remove or insert the electrical leads unless the power supply is turned off. Start with the power off and the voltage and current turned all the way down to zero before connecting the leads (red to red and black to black), then turn on and bring voltage and current up slowly to desired level. Reverse this procedure to disconnect the gel. If a gel is disconnected before turning off the power, considerable electrical energy remains in the power unit and can discharge through the sockets even though the unit is turned off.**
3. **Always remove leads one at a time with the other hand free or on a nonconducting surface. Using both hands can create a very dangerous shunt of current across the chest and through the heart if you contact a bare wire.**

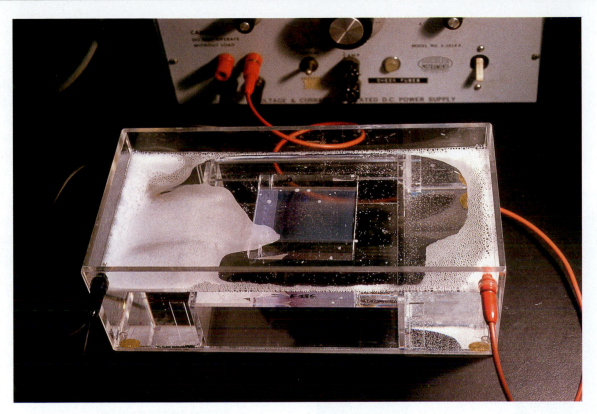

Figure 17.2   Electrophoresis of a gel

D.   Blot Transfer

Transfer of the proteins from the gel to the membrane can be carried out by placing the membrane on top of the gel and moving the proteins to it either electrophoretically using a special blot transfer electrophoresis unit, or by diffusion by "wicking." The second method takes longer but requires no expensive equipment.

Materials for Part D:
- ☐ gloves
- ☐ 2 large sponges
- ☐ 1 nitrocellulose membrane
- ☐ blotting papers
- ☐ glass plate
- ☐ transfer buffer
- ☐ glass casserole dish

Procedure:

1. Wear gloves throughout the following steps to avoid contaminating the gel or the membrane with proteins from your hands. Cut a piece of nitrocellulose membrane and 4 sheets of blotting paper to the exact size of your gel. Also cut a 3-inch stack of blotting paper or paper towels to the size of your gel. Soak the membrane and 4 sheets of blotting paper in transfer buffer for 15 to 20 minutes.

2. Build the transfer sandwich as follows. Completely saturate the sponges in transfer buffer and place in the casserole dish. Stack 2 pieces of the wet blotting paper on top of the sponges. Carefully remove the gel from the electrophoresis unit and lay on top of the blotting papers with the well side down. Place the membrane on the top of this stack (on the backside of the gel), followed by the remaining 2 pieces of wet blotting paper. Smooth each layer with your (gloved) finger to remove air bubbles between layers. Place the 3-inch stack of dry papers on top, and cover the whole stack with a glass plate. Weight down

the stack *lightly* with an object such as a book or a bottle of buffer, just enough weight to ensure even contact of the layers (fig. 17.3).

3. Add transfer buffer to the dish to a level halfway up the sides of the two sponges. Let sit from 1 hour to overnight at room temperature.

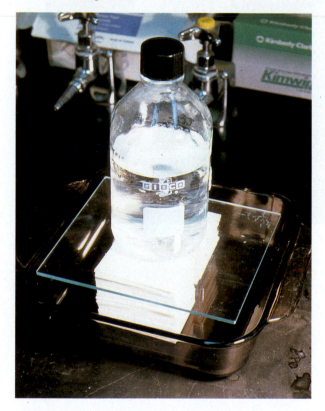

Figure 17.3   Western blot transfer

E.   Antibody Incubations

The antibody label used in this exercise is the chromogenic enzyme **horse radish peroxidase** (HRPO), which catalyzes the reaction shown in figure 17.4. After all antibody incubations are completed, the membrane is soaked in a solution of the enzyme's substrate (4-chloro-1-napthol). A purple spot will be seen on the membrane in every place where an antigen has bound the primary antibody followed by binding of the enzyme-labeled secondary antibody. Unless an antigen which reacts with the primary antibody was present in the protein sample, the membrane will remain colorless throughout.

Materials for Part E:

- ☐ gloves
- ☐ 2 casserole dishes
- ☐ blocking solution (1% gelatin or 10% nonfat dry milk in PBS)
- ☐ antibody against human serum proteins (produced in a rabbit)
- ☐ HRPO-labeled antibodies (IgG) against rabbit antibody
- ☐ phosphate buffered saline (PBS)
- ☐ 4-chloro-1-napthol substrate tablets
- ☐ methanol
- ☐ 3% hydrogen peroxide solution
- ☐ 37°C incubator

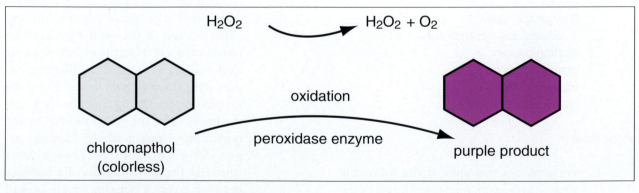

Figure 17.4   Reaction catalyzed by HRPO enzyme

Procedure:

1. Wear gloves throughout the following steps. Disassemble the blotting "sandwich" and remove the membrane. The gel and blotting paper can be discarded. Allow the membrane to air dry for about 30 minutes at 37°C or until completely dry (the membrane will start to curl at the edges).

2. Pour out the transfer buffer and rinse the glass dish with water. Place the membrane in the dish and cover it with blocking solution. Incubate the blot for 1 hour at room temperature with gentle rocking. After this point the blot may be stored in the refrigerator until the next lab period if necessary.

3. Dilute the primary antibody to human serum proteins by adding 250 µl of antibody to 50 mls of blocking solution. Pour the old blocking solution off the blot and add the antibody solution to the blot in the glass staining dish. Incubate the blot for 2 hours to overnight with gentle mechanical rotation.

4. Pour off the antibody solution. Wash the blot 5 times in 50 mls of PBS for 5 minutes each wash.

5. While the blot is washing, dilute the HRPO-labeled antiserum by adding 250 µl of antiserum to 50 ml of PBS.

6. Pour off the last wash buffer and add the diluted secondary antibody to the blot. Incubate 1 hour with gentle rocking.

7. Pour off the antibody solution and wash the blot 5 times in 50 mls PBS for 5 minutes each wash. Do not let the membrane dry. Leave it in the PBS until you are ready for the next step.

8. While the blot is washing, prepare the substrate solution by dissolving 3 mg of 4-chloro-1-naphthol in 1 ml of methanol. Dilute this solution to a final volume of 10 mls with PBS, and filter through a Whatman #1 or equivalent filter to remove the precipitate that forms. Then add 20 µl of 3% hydrogen peroxide to the filtered solution.

9. Pour the last wash solution off the blot, then transfer the blot to a small dish containing the substrate solution. Gently rock the blot until purple bands appear (usually about 30 minutes).

10. Remove the blot from the substrate and rinse it in water to stop the color development. The blot may now be stored indefinitely if protected from light. Record your results by drawing a picture of the membrane in figure 17.5 below, noting the lane number and migration distance of each protein detected.

Figure 17.5   Results of Western Blot

Additional Reading:

1. Harlow, E., and D. Lane. 1988. Antibodies: A Laboratory Manual. Cold Spring Harbor, New York: Cold Spring Harbor Laboratory.

2. Voller, A., and D. Bidwell, eds. 1981. Immunoassays for the 80's. Baltimore, Maryland: University Park Press.

3. Richardson, J. S. 1981. The anatomy and taxonomy of protein structure. Adv. Protein Chem. 34:167.

4. Hames, B. D., and D. Richwood. 1981. Gel Electrophoresis of Proteins. Oxford: IRL Press.

Key terms:

Western blot
immunoblot
"tag" or "label"
chromogenic enzyme
radioisotope
primary antibody
secondary antibody

Questions:

1. How did the term "Western" blot originate?

2. Why is nonspecific protein binding a problem and how does the use of gelatin solve this problem?

3. How many different proteins were you able to detect in your serum sample? Can you identify any of these based on molecular weight?

18 Enzyme-Linked ImmunoSorbent Assay (ELISA)

Enzyme-labeled antibody can be used in several applications including the Western blot, direct and indirect staining of antigen prepared as smears or tissue sections of specimens on microscope slides, and in the frequently used microtiter procedure for quantifying antibody known as the ELISA. The ELISA technique is an extremely sensitive method for detecting antigens or antibodies. Quantities as low as 1 nanogram/ml of protein can be detected.

The ELISA procedure takes advantage of the fact that most proteins will adhere to plastic. Thus, a specific antigen is placed in the wells of a plastic microtiter plate and allowed to bind (fig. 18.1). Any plastic remaining uncovered by antigen is then coated by a blocking protein (any protein unrelated to the test components) to avoid subsequent nonspecific binding of antibody in the next step. Now a sample of antibody or antiserum is added to the wells, which will bind if the appropriate antigen has bound in the first step. The plate is washed to remove unbound antibody. The presence of any bound antibody remaining in the wells can then be detected by the use of a secondary enzyme conjugate. The conjugate consists of either antibody against the immunoglobulin class of the first antibody (the theory is similar to that for the western blot), or sometimes a protein called protein-A derived from the cell wall of the bacterium *Staphylococcus aureus* which has the unique characteristic of binding to immunoglobulins of a variety of species. Finally, the conjugate, if bound to the wells, can be detected by addition of the enzyme substrate and the subsequent color change observed (fig. 18.2).

Enzyme conjugates have several advantages over other types of conjugates like fluorescent or radioactive conjugates. With fluorescent conjugates, the fluorescence gradually disappears due to quenching on exposure to light, the reagents are unstable, expensive equipment is necessary to view the results, and interpretation of the results can be somewhat subjective. Radioactive conjugates have the obvious disadvantage of being hazardous. The use of chromogenic enzyme labels in antibody conjugates eliminates these problems, and the results obtained can easily be read with the naked eye, or spectrophotometrically if precise quantitative measurements are desired.

Materials:

- [ ] 96-well microtiter plates with flat-bottomed wells
- [ ] 10-ml pipettes
- [ ] solutions of three different antigens (1% in PBS)
- [ ] antiserum
- [ ] 24 test tubes containing 0.5 mls saline
- [ ] sample of known antibody against the antigen (control antiserum)
- [ ] blocking buffer (1% gelatin in PBS)
- [ ] PBS-Tween 20
- [ ] conjugate (protein A-Horse radish peroxidase)
- [ ] substrate solution (5-aminosalysilic acid)
- [ ] 2 squirt bottles
- [ ] 200 µl automatic pipette and tips
- [ ] 37°C incubator

Procedure:

1. *The following is to be done the day before or during the previous exercise.*
   Choose 4 wells on a 96-well, flat-bottom microtiter plate to designate as control wells (the first 4 wells of row A are most convenient). Label these wells 1A, 2A, 3A, and 4A. Using a 10-ml pipette, add 2 drops of the first antigen solution to each well of rows B and C, and to control wells 2A, 3A, and 4A. Do not add antigen to control well 1A. Add the sec-

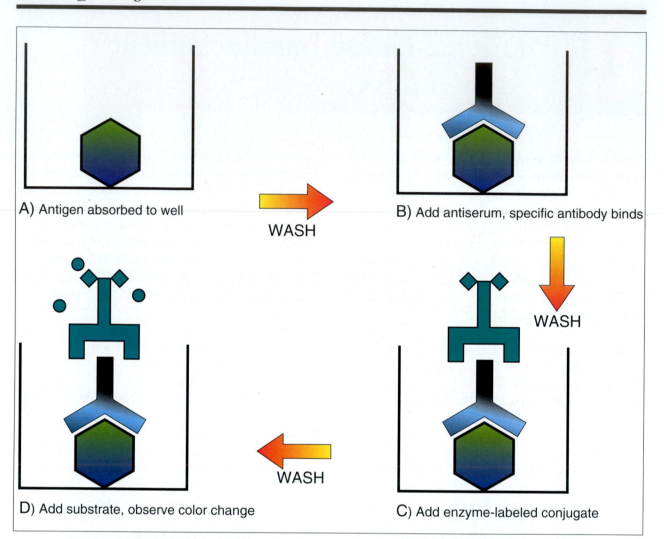

A) Antigen absorbed to well

WASH

B) Add antiserum, specific antibody binds

WASH

D) Add substrate, observe color change

WASH

C) Add enzyme-labeled conjugate

Figure 18.1 ELISA Procedure. The ELISA procedure has been applied in many situations, including the detection of antibody to the AIDS virus, and may be one of the most popular and versatile immunological assays available. You will use the assay in this exercise to determine the titer and specificity of an antiserum for three different antigens You may also use this assay to detect antibody production by hybridomas, and to determine the purity of an affinity-filtered preparation of antibody in other exercises. The conjugate used in this exercise is protein-A labeled with horse radish peroxidase.

ond antigen to wells of rows D and E in the same manner, and add the third antigen to rows F and G. Cover the plate with plastic wrap and allow to sit overnight (or up to 3 weeks) at 4°C.

2. Dump out the antigen solutions by inverting the plate over the sink, then blotting dry on a stack of paper towels. *Completely* fill each well with blocking buffer from a squirt bottle. Cover the plate and incubate at 37°C for 15 minutes.

3. Invert the plate over a sink to discard the blocking solution, then blot dry.

4. Wash the wells by filling them with PBS-Tween from a squirt bottle. Dump out the plate and repeat the wash twice more. Blot the plate on paper towels.

5. Prepare two-fold dilutions of the antiserum by serially transferring 0.5 mls antiserum through 24 0.5-ml saline dilution blanks. This will give you 0.5

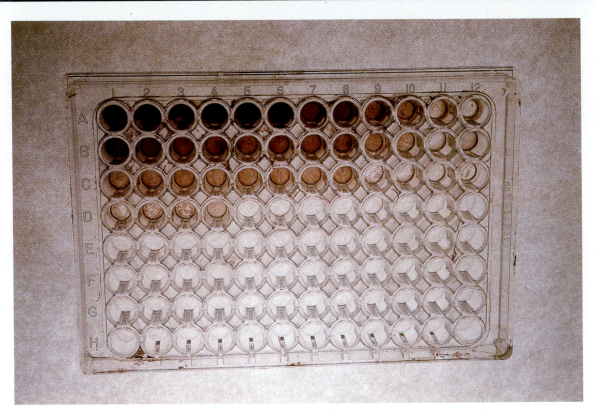

Figure 18.2   Color changes of substrate seen in an ELISA plate

ml of each dilution, enough for use with each of the three antigens. Being *very careful* not to splatter or misplace drops, add 100 μl of each antiserum dilution to the wells of rows B and C of the ELISA plate.
Use a new pipette tip for each well. Repeat for the other two antigens. Add the control antiserum to control wells 1A, 3A, and 4A (not to well 2A). Cover the plate with plastic wrap and incubate for 30 minutes at 37°C.

6. Wash and drain the plate 3 times with PBS-Tween as in step 4.

7. Using a 10-ml pipette, add 2 drops of conjugate to every well used except control well 3A. Cover the plate and incubate for 30 minutes at 37°C.

8. Wash and drain the plates 3 times in water, 3 times in PBS-tween, and 3 times again in water and blot as in step 3.

9. Using a 10-ml pipette, add 2 drops of freshly prepared substrate solution to each well used except control well 4A. Cover the plate and incubate for 15 to 30 minutes at 37°C. Wells which contain bound antibody will develop a dark brown color. The color may vary with the antiserum dilution, but any well having more color than the negative controls is considered positive. Make sure all the control wells are negative. Record your results in Table 18.1.

Table 18.1 ELISA Results ("+" indicates a color change took place)

	1	2	3	4	5	6	7	8	9	10	11	12
A												
B												
C												
D												
E												
F												
G												
H												

Key Terms:

chromogenic enzyme conjugate
protein-A

Questions:

1. What is the purpose of each of the control wells? Should they show any change in color?

2. What is the purpose of the gelatin blocking solution?

Additional Reading:

1. Engvall, E., and P. Perlmann. 1971. Enzyme Linked Immunosorbent Assay (ELISA): quantitative assay of immunoglobulin G. Immunochemistry 8:1175.

2. Galen, R. S., et al. 1976. The enzyme multiplied immunoassay. Lancet 2:852.

3. Avrameas, S., et al. 1983. Immunoenzymatic Techniques. Amsterdam: Elsevier Science Publishers.

19 Indirect Fluorescent Antibody Testing

The ability to bind chemical markers to antibodies without interfering with antigen-binding ability makes antibodies very useful staining reagents for the specific detection of antigens. Several different types of chemical markers, also known as "tags," can be covalently coupled to antibodies. These include radioactive isotopes, enzymes, and fluorescent compounds. The tagged antibody is called a conjugate, and allows visual detection of the antigen to which it binds.

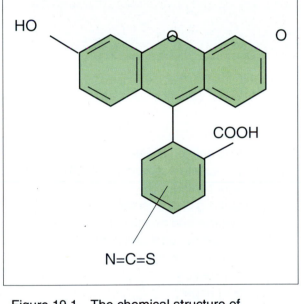

Figure 19.1   The chemical structure of fluorescein

The technique of immunofluorescence utilizes specific antibody tagged with fluorochromes, compounds which absorb ultraviolet light and then emit light in the visible range as fluorescence. One of the most commonly used fluorescent tags is fluorescein (fig. 19.1), which emits a bright, apple-green flourescence under UV light (fig. 19.2).

As with the Western blot detection system, immunofluorescence can be used in either a direct or an indirect assay. In the direct assay, fluorescent-tagged antibody directed against the antigen to be detected is applied directly to the sample. The sample may be bacterial cells, a tissue sample, or viral-infected cells, and the conjugate would be something like fluorescein-labeled anti-bacterial or anti-viral antibody. If the antigen of interest is present in the sample, the conjugate will bind to the antigen, resulting in fluorescence on the sample that can be seen under an ultraviolet microscope.

In the indirect assay, serum (usually from a human patient) is applied to the sample. In the second step, fluorescent-labeled antibody directed against human immunoglobulin (Ig) is applied to the sample. The anti-human Ig is usually produced by immunizing a rabbit or goat with human immunoglobulin. If the serum contained specific antibody against the antigen, these antibodies will bind to the sample in the first step. Application of the conjugate in the second step allows detection of bound antibody. Indirect immunofluorescence is often used to determine whether a patient is producing antibody against a particular infectious agent in order to confirm a diagnosis. As with the agglutination assay, dilutions of the serum can be tested to demonstrate the four-fold increase in antibody titer that would confirm illness with the suspected pathogen.

In this exercise, you will use prepared antigen slides and your own serum to determine whether you have antibody to the antigens provided in your own blood. The slides have wells which contain viral-infected cells. When a virus infects a cell, it expresses its own antigens on the cell surface. It is these antigens which can be detected by serum antibodies. The slides have been fixed, so the virus is no longer infectious. The viruses

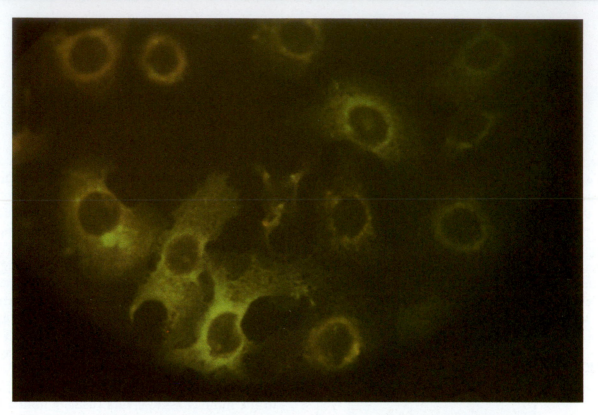

Figure 19.2   This cell culture was infected with Rubella virus and has been stained in the indirect fluorescent antibody procedure. The infected cells fluoresce an apple green color.

that have been chosen are ones to which you or some of your classmates are probably immune, either because of childhood illness or vaccination. Therefore, you should be successful in demonstrating a positive result for antibody.

Materials:
- ☐ sterile lancets
- ☐ 70% ethanol
- ☐ cotton balls
- ☐ fingertip bandages
- ☐ 3 small glass tubes or Eppendorf tubes
- ☐ automatic pipette and tips
- ☐ viral antigen slides
- ☐ phosphate buffered saline (PBS)
- ☐ squirt bottle
- ☐ staining dish or small jar
- ☐ positive and negative control sera
- ☐ conjugate (goat anti-human IgG-fluorescein)
- ☐ petri plates
- ☐ filter paper
- ☐ bibulous paper
- ☐ buffered glycerol mounting medium
- ☐ microscope coverslips (22 × 50 mm)
- ☐ fluorescent microscope

⚠ *Safety Tips:*
1.   **Do not exchange lancets.**
2.   **Handle only your own serum.**
3.   **Dispose of lancets, cotton balls, bandages, and the like only in the container provided for that purpose.**
4.   **Wear gloves if sharing a slide with another individual.**

116

Procedure:

1. Have a sterile lancet and a clean, dry cotton ball ready. Clean your left "ring" finger tip with an alcohol-soaked cotton ball and let it air-dry.

2. Puncture your finger with the lancet, trying to strike at the side of the finger tip to avoid the calloused skin in the center.

3. Discard the first drop of blood by wiping it away with the cotton ball.

4. Allow the blood to drip into a small glass tube or Eppendorf tube. Try to obtain approximately 0.5 mls (about 5 to 10 large drops).

5. Let the blood sit for 20 to 30 minutes. Meanwhile, make sure the viral antigen slides have been allowed to come to room temperature if they have been stored in the refrigerator.

6. Place 90 ml of PBS in each of two small tubes to use as dilution blanks. Withdraw 10 ml serum from the tube of blood and transfer it to a dilution blank. Transfer a second 10 ml from the first dilution blank to the second. You now have a 1:10 dilution and a 1:100 dilution of test serum.

7. Making sure to change pipette tips between each sample, place 10 µl of each serum dilution on a well of the antigen plate. If you still have more serum, you may also place 10 µl of undilute serum on a third well. Place 10 µl of a positive control serum and 10 µl of a negative control serum on wells 4 and 5. Record the placement of your samples. (Note— two individuals may share one 8-well slide. Only one set of control sera is needed per slide).

8. Make sure the samples completely cover the wells. If not, use a clean pipette tip to carefully spread the serum over each well. Do not scrape the surface of the wells.

9. Place the slide in a petri plate containing a damp piece of filter paper, and incubate at room temperature for 30 minutes.

10. Rinse the slide with PBS from a squirt bottle. Do not squirt the PBS directly at the wells as you might dislodge the cells. Instead, let the buffer run down the slide to rinse.

11. Place the slide in a staining dish or small jar filled with PBS. Let sit for 15 minutes with gentle agitation.

12. Remove the slide from the PBS and let air dry. You may blot excess moisture carefully with bibulous paper, but be careful not to scrape the wells.

13. Cover each of the 5 wells well with 10 µls of conjugate. Incubate the slide in the petri plate for 30 minutes at room temperature.

14. Repeat washing steps 11 through 13.

15. Place four small drops of buffered glycerol on the middle of the slide between the wells (do not place directly over the wells). Cover the slide with a coverslip and press down slightly. The glycerol should flow into the wells.

16. View the slide under the fluorescent microscope (fig 19.3). Compare the amount of fluorescence between the samples and the controls. Fluorescence of the 1:10 and/or 1:100 indicates the presence of specific antibody in the serum. Fluorescence of only the undiluted

serum may be nonspecific. Table 19.1 lists the expected results for positive IFA reactions on a variety of different viral antigen slides. The slides may be stored in the dark at 4°C.

Key Terms:

fluorochrome
immunofluorescence

Questions:

1. What is the difference between the direct and the indirect tests in fluorescent antibody testing?

Additional Reading:

1. Coons, A. H., and M. H. Kaplan. 1950. Localization of antigen in tissue cells. II. Improvements in a method for the detection of antigen by means of fluorescent antibody. J. Exp. Med. 91:1–13.

2. Burrell, R. 1974. Experimental Immunology. Minneapolis, Minnesota: Burgess Publishing Co.

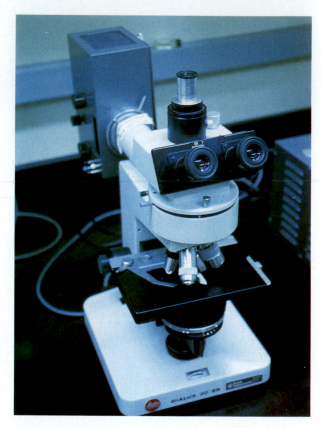

Figure 19.3   A fluorescent microscope

Table 19.1   Appearance of the Positive Reaction for Several Viral Indirect Fluorescent Antibody Tests.

Virus	Appearance of Stained cells
Measles	Bright apple-green fluorescence in the cytoplasm of infected cells
Mumps	Bright apple-green fluorescence of round inclusions in the cytoplasm of infected cells
Rubella	Bright yellow-green fluorescence of the cytoplasm of infected cells
Varicella (chicken pox)	Bright yellow-green fluorescence in the cytoplasm and/or nucleus of infected cells

20 Murder Mystery -- A Forensics Problem

This exercise is a simple example of how an immunological assay might be used to solve a forensics problem. You will be given a blood-stained cloth, and will be asked to determine whether the blood is of human or animal origin by using the Ouchterlony test.

Materials:
- ☐ blood-stained cloth
- ☐ scissors
- ☐ beaker
- ☐ 5 mls saline
- ☐ Ouchterlony plate: 3 petri plates each containing 15 ml of 1% agarose + 2% PEG 6000 in PBS containing 0.05% NaN_2
- ☐ antisera against several animal species, including human
- ☐ 1% saline solutions of serum albumin from each species to be tested
- ☐ Pasteur pipettes
- ☐ tape or small plastic bag with sponge

Procedure:

1. With a scissors, cut out just the portion of the cloth that is stained with blood. Place the cloth in a beaker containing 5 mls of saline.

2. Let the cloth soak for a few minutes, then rinse out as much of the blood as possible into the saline.

3. Prepare one Ouchterlony plate for each antiserum type to be tested in the same way as in exercise 13 by punching the template and removing the agar plugs from the wells.

4. Fill the center well of each plate with one of the various samples of anti-species antisera. The wells should be completely filled, but not overfilled.

5. Add the blood-saline mixture and each of the known protein solutions separately to the outer wells of each plate.

6. Seal the plate with tape or place the plate in a plastic bag with a wet sponge to keep the plate moist. Incubate the plate at room temperature for 48 hours.

7. Look for lines of precipitation to determine the identity of the blood sample.

Questions:

1. What are the controls used for this exercise?

2. Why were albumins chosen for known protein samples?

Additional Reading:

1. Ouchterlony, O. 1949. Antigen-antibody reactions in gels. Acta Pathol. Microbiol. Scand. 26:507.

2. Williams, C. A., and M. W. Chase, eds. 1971. Methods in Immunology and Immunochemistry, vol. 3. New York: Academic Press.

Section 3

Advanced Exercises in Immunology

21 Preparation of Hybridomas for Monoclonal Antibody

When an antigen is introduced into an animal, B-cells are stimulated to produce antibody directed against the antigen. Each B-cell that recognizes a presented antigen will proliferate by dividing into identical **clones** of the original cell, with each of the clones producing identical antibody. If the antigen is complex and has many epitopes, many clones of B-cells, each originating from different B-cells responding to different epitopes, will be produced. This is termed a **polyclonal response**. The serum harvested from such an animal will contain a mixture of antibodies of different antigenic specificities and binding affinities. Because of this heterogeneity, polyclonal antisera have limited usefulness in many immunological applications. For example, it is frequently necessary to use species- or even strain-specific antibody for definitive identification of bacteria in clinical laboratories, but even antisera produced by injecting an animal with a pure culture may contain cross-reacting antibodies because similar microorganisms often share some antigenic determinants. Several techniques may be employed to make an antiserum more specific, such as adsorption of cross-reactive antibody or affinity chromatography, but these methods provide only a limited amount of antibody.

The development of hybridoma technology by Kohler and Milstein in 1975 led to the ability to produce large quantities of monoclonal antibody, or antibody produced by cells originating from a single clone. The **monoclonal antibody** preparation, containing molecules which are all structurally identical and therefore have the identical antigen specificity and binding affinity, provides many advantages over the use of conventional antisera.

Production of monoclonal antibody (figure 21.1) involves fusing spleen cells (B-cells) from an immunized animal with **myeloma** cells (tumor cells of B-cell lineage), and then growing the fused cells (**hybridomas**) in 96-well tissue culture plates. The hybridomas possess both the ability to produce antibody and the immortality of the myeloma cell. They can be cultured indefinitely and tested to determine which clone is producing the desired antibody. The clone can then be cultured in large quantities for harvesting of monoclonal antibody.

The use of monoclonal antibody has resulted in tremendous advances in biological and medical research. Monoclonal antibodies are being produced commercially for immunodiagnosis and are also being studied for their use in the diagnosis and treatment of cancer.

The procedure for monoclonal antibody production requires about two months. All parts of the procedure must be carried out with *strict* attention to sterile technique and within a laminar flow hood. The following steps are involved:

A. immunization of mice.

B. culture of myeloma cells.

C. fusion procedure.

D. feeding hybridomas with selective media.

E. ELISA to evaluate specific antibody production.

F. cloning by limiting dilution.

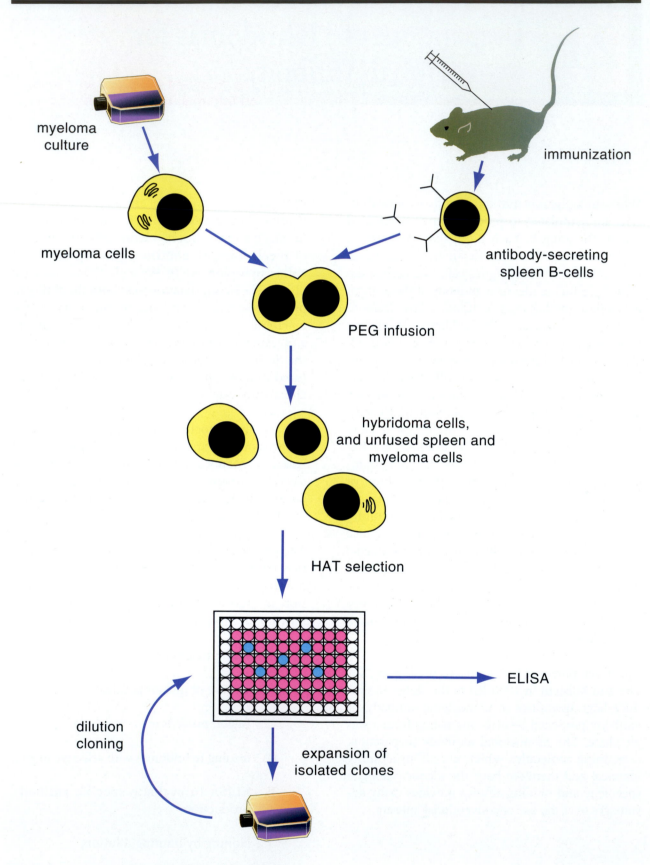

myeloma
culture

immunization

myeloma cells

antibody-secreting
spleen B-cells

PEG infusion

hybridoma cells,
and unfused spleen and
myeloma cells

HAT selection

ELISA

dilution
cloning

expansion of
isolated clones

Figure 21.1   Production of monoclonal antibody.

A.   Immunization of Mice

Materials for Part A:

☐ female Balb/c mouse, about 6 weeks old
☐ solution of soluble protein antigen in saline (1 mg/ml)
☐ complete Freund's adjuvant (CFA)
☐ incomplete Freund's adjuvant (IFA)
☐ double-hub syringes
☐ 25 gauge needle
☐ 1 ml syringes

Table 21.1   Experimental Schedule

Day	Procedure:
1	intraperitoneal immunization
5–7	start myeloma culture
14	intraperitoneal booster
18	dilute myeloma culture to 1×10^5 cells/ml
19	cell fusion
20	begin feeding cells HAT
26–29	ELISA, expand hybridomas, feed with HT
45	begin feeding cells growth medium
45+	cloning
45+	final ELISA

⚠ *Safety Tip:*

The adjuvant mixture can cause an inflammatory reaction if accidentally inoculated. Do not splatter into the eyes—wear goggles during use.

Procedure:

1. Prepare the antigen/CFA mixture (1 to 1 ratio) as described in exercise 9, part 2A.

2. Inject the mouse in the peritoneal cavity with 0.1 ml of antigen emulsion to give a dose of 50 µg protein. Use a 25-gauge needle for injection. The injection technique should be demonstrated by your instructor (also see fig. 2.1). To inject the mouse, hold it at the base of the tail with your right hand (if you are right-handed), and let it cling to the top of its cage as you grasp the back of the neck with your left hand. You must pinch together all the loose skin right behind the ears between your thumb and the knuckle of your index finger so that the mouse is immobilized and cannot turn its head around to bite. Then lay the mouse across your hand with its back against your closed fingers, and clamp the tail and left leg of the mouse under your pinky. Insert the needle with the bevel facing up about 1/4 inch into the mouse's left lower abdomen. Inject the 0.1 mls of antigen mixture.

3. After 14 days (see schedule in table 21.1), prepare a second emulsion of the antigen, this time in incomplete Freund's adjuvant (as in exercise 9, part 2A). Boost the mouse with one 0.1 ml intraperitoneal injection of this emulsion.

4. Three to five days after the last boost the spleen should be obtained for fusion.

B. Culture of Myeloma cells

The myeloma cell is a cancerous (transformed) cell of B-cell lineage, but because B-cells become transformed in a random manner it is not possible to direct their antigen specificity. Unlike normal spleen cells, however, the myeloma cell will grow indefinitely, and when fused with immune spleen cells allows the resulting hybridoma to be cultured *in vitro*. Two of the most commonly used myeloma cell lines are SP/2, and NS-1 from the balb/c mouse. The myeloma cultures must be prepared well in advance of the fusion date, and should be "split" (diluted in fresh medium) the day before the fusion to make sure they are in log-phase growth.

Materials for Part B:

- ☐ vial or culture of myeloma cells (NS-1 or SP/2)
- ☐ Myeloma growth medium: RPMI-1640 + glutamine + 10% fetal bovine serum (FBS) + gentamicin (50 µg/ml) or penicillin(100 U/ml)/streptomycin (100 µg/ml)
- ☐ tissue culture flasks (25 cm^2)
- ☐ sterile 10-ml cotton-plugged pipettes
- ☐ sterile 1-ml cotton-plugged pipettes
- ☐ small bottle of 70% ethanol
- ☐ 37°C CO^2 incubator
- ☐ 37°C water bath
- ☐ clinical centrifuge

Procedure:

1. Begin growing the myelomas about 2 weeks prior to fusion. They will need about one week to recuperate from frozen storage. To reconstitute frozen cells, place the bottom of the cryovial containing the cells in a 37°C water bath, but do not submerge the vial completely. Shake the vial in the water gently for a few minutes until thawed.

2. In the laminar flow hood, decontaminate the outside of the vial by wiping with ethanol, then resuspend the cells gently and transfer to a centrifuge tube containing 9 mls of growth medium. Centrifuge 5 minutes at $500 \times g$.

3. Discard the supernatant and resuspend the cells in a flask with 10 mls growth medium. Grow the cells in growth medium at 37°C in 5 to 7% CO$_2$. Always make sure the cap of the tissue culture flask is loosened before incubating cells in the CO$_2$ incubator. If the cells become crowded enough to almost completely cover the bottom of the flask, you will have to shake the cells loose (make sure the cap is tightly shut when you do this), and transfer half the culture to a new flask with an equal volume of fresh growth medium. The culture becomes crowded and needs to be "split" in this manner when the cells reach a density of 1×10^6 cells/ml (fig. 21.2).

4. The day before the fusion, shake the myeloma cells loose in their flask and dilute 1 to 2 in an equal volume of fresh growth medium, as described above.

C. Cell Fusion

Certain viruses have outer lipoprotein envelopes that are similar to the plasma membranes of animal cells, and have been used to fuse cells together. The mechanism of fusion seems to involve glycoproteins in the viral envelope, although this isn't proven.

Sendai virus was originally used to fuse B-cells with myeloma cells, but now polyethylene glycol (PEG) is used instead of the virus. The exact mechanism of PEG fusion is not well understood, but it appears that PEG promotes the close apposition of cell membranes while other additives in the commercial preparation actually stimulate fusion. This may explain why different brands or lots of PEG can have highly variable fusion efficiencies. Because PEG is toxic to cells, exposure during the fusion process must be limited as much as possible. Alternatives to PEG as a fusion agent are currently under study.

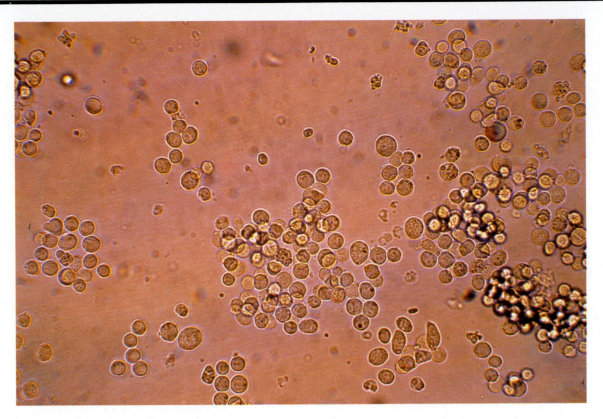

Figure 21.2   A heavily-grown culture of myeloma cells.

Following fusion, the new hybridomas are cultured in growth medium containing extra serum and a "feeder-conditioned medium" supplement. This is medium taken from a culture of macrophage or thymocyte cells, and contains components which help the fragile hybridomas grow.

Materials for Part C:
- ☐ immunized mouse
- ☐ mouse jar with anesthetic and cotton balls
- ☐ dissection tray, scissors, and forceps
- ☐ 70% ethanol in a squirt bottle
- ☐ jar containing 95% ethanol
- ☐ myeloma cell culture (leave in incubator until needed)
- ☐ sterile petri plate containing a piece of stainless steel mesh
- ☐ 80 mls wash medium (RPMI without serum), held at 37°C
- ☐ red blood cell lysing buffer
- ☐ 10 mls hybridoma growth medium (RPMI + 15% FBS + gentamicin (50 µg/ml) or penicillin(100 U/ml)/streptomycin (100 µg/ml) + 10% feeder-conditioned medium)
- ☐ 10 mls HAT medium (hybridoma growth medium + HAT additive)
- ☐ 3 50-ml sterile centrifuge tubes
- ☐ hemocytometer and trypan blue dye
- ☐ sterile tissue paper or gauze
- ☐ 1 ml PEG solution (50% pre-screened PEG 1500 in RPMI)
- ☐ gloves
- ☐ sterile 1-ml cotton-plugged pipettes
- ☐ sterile 10-ml cotton-plugged pipettes
- ☐ cell culture plate (96-well, flat-bottom)
- ☐ small 37°C water bath and ice bucket
- ☐ clinical centrifuge

⚠ ***Safety Tips:***

1.   **Avoid breathing anesthetic vapors.**
2.   **Be careful not to let ethanol drip down onto your hand when flaming dissection tools, and do not place hot dissection tools directly into the ethanol or touch the ethanol-doused mouse.**
3.   **If an ethanol fire does occur, don't panic or use water, but simply smother the fire with a beaker or towel.**
4.   **Wear protective gloves during handling of the PEG—it is toxic.**
5.   **Wear protective gloves during handling of the HAT medium—the aminopterin component is toxic.**

Procedure:

Myeloma cells are fragile—do not process until just before the fusion. Prepare the spleen cells first.

1.   Euthanize a mouse by placing it in a jar or coffee can which contains a couple large cotton balls soaked in anesthetic. Close the jar tightly for 5 minutes.

2.   Use careful aseptic technique for the following procedures. Wet down the euthanized mouse with 70% ethanol. Sterilize a scissors and forceps by dipping them in 95% ethanol and passing them quickly through the Bunsen burner flame to burn off the alcohol. Pull up the skin of the abdomen with the sterile forceps and cut through the abdomen longitudinally with the scissors. Cut and fold back the skin of the abdomen to expose the internal organs.

3.   Dip and flame the scissors and forceps again, then locate the spleen. The spleen is a long, flat, reddish organ lying directly under the stomach. Remove the spleen with the forceps (you may need to cut it free from connecting tissues) and place it in the sterile petri plate containing the steel mesh (fig. 21.3).

4.   Add 10 ml of wash medium to the petri plate. Mince the spleen as finely as possible on the screen using sterile (alcohol-flamed) scissors. Dip the mesh repeatedly into the wash medium to disperse the cells.

5.   Transfer the spleen cell suspension into a 50-ml centrifuge tube. If large chunks of debris are present, let these settle for a few minutes, before transferring the suspension to the centrifuge tube. Discard the debris.

6.   Centrifuge the spleen cell suspension at $500 \times g$ for 5 minutes. Also add 10 mls of the wash medium to the 10-ml myeloma culture and shake the cells loose from the flask.

7.   After the centrifuge has come to a stop, remove the supernatant from the spleen cell pellet and discard. Lyse red blood cells in the spleen cell suspension by adding 10 mls lysing buffer to the tube. Let sit on ice for 8 minutes, then slowly fill the tube with wash medium. While the red blood cells are lysing, transfer the 20 mls of myeloma cells to a separate centrifuge tube. Centrifuge both cell suspensions at the same time ($500 \times g$ for 5 minutes).

8.   Wash each cell pellet once more in 10 mls wash medium.

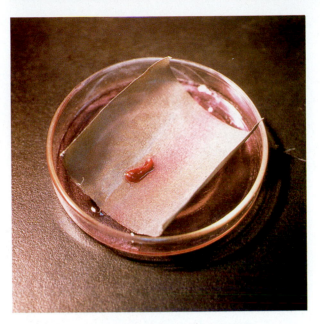

Figure 21.3   A spleen placed on a piece of steel mesh.

9. After the final centrifuge spins, remove and discard the supernatants from both cell pellets. Resuspend each pellet in 10 mls wash medium, and combine the two cell populations in the same tube. Centrifuge at $500 \times g$ for 5 minutes.

10. After the centrifuge has come to a stop, remove the supernatant from the cell pellet but *do not resuspend the pellet*. Aspirate as much of the supernatant as possible, then drain the tube on a piece of sterile tissue paper or gauze.

11. Loosen the pellet with a slight tap of the tube, and place the tube in a 37°C water bath. A small water bath for inside the hood can be prepared by placing a beaker containing 37°C water (taken from a larger water bath) inside a larger beaker also containing 37°C water (fig. 21.4). The inner beaker will hold its temperature long enough to carry out the fusion. Slowly add 1 ml of PEG solution drop by drop, over a 1 minute period, while gently stirring the cells with the tip of a sterile 1-ml pipette. Stir for an additional 1 minute at 37°C. Imme-

diately add 1 ml of warm wash medium, drop by drop, over the next 1 minute while stirring continuously, then add 9 mls drop by drop over 2 to 3 minutes.

12. Centrifuge the cells at $500 \times g$ for 5 minutes. Meanwhile, warm the growth medium in the water bath.

13. Discard the supernatant and resuspend the cells by gently adding 10 mls of hybridoma growth medium. The fused cells are very fragile. Do not shake the tube or pipette up and down to resuspend, but stir gently with a pipette to loosen the pellet, then let sit for a few minutes until the cells disperse.

14. Using a 10-ml pipette, add two drops of the cell suspension to all except the outermost wells of the 96-well microtiter plate. Incubate at 37°C in 5 to 7% CO_2 overnight.

15. The next day, add 2 drops of HAT medium to each filled well with a 10-ml pipette (see part D).

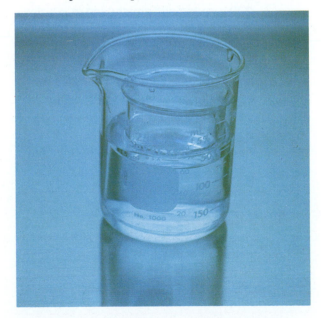

Figure 21.4   A small "water bath" for inside the hood.

D.   Feeding the Hybridomas

Isolation of the desired hybridoma clones from the mixed culture requires that all unfused spleen cells and myeloma cells be eliminated. The spleen cells will simply die out because they cannot live long in culture.

Myeloma cell types SP/2 and NS-1 are mutants which lack the gene for the enzyme **hypoxanthine phosphoribosyl transferase**, which means they cannot utilize hypoxanthine to manufacture purines and pyrimidines via the salvage pathway. Therefore, by growing the cell fusion mixture in a growth medium containing three special ingredients, hypoxanthine, **aminopterin**, and thymidine (HAT medium), unfused myelomas can be eliminated. The aminopterin is a folic acid analog which blocks de novo synthesis of nucleotides, thus preventing the cells from making their own purines and pyrimidines from scratch. Because myeloma cells also cannot utilize the hypoxanthine from the medium, they will die. The hybrid cells, however, possess a functional enzyme obtained from the normal spleen cells, and can utilize hypoxanthine and thymidine to survive.

Materials for Part D:

- [ ] 200 μl automatic pipette and sterile tips
- [ ] sterile 10-ml cotton-plugged pipettes
- [ ] HAT medium
- [ ] HT medium
- [ ] myeloma growth medium (RPMI + 10% FBS + gentamicin (50 μg/ml) or penicillin (100 U/ml)/streptomycin (100 μg/ml))
- [ ] cell culture plates (24-well, flat-bottom)
- [ ] cell culture flasks (25 cm^2)

⚠ *Safety Tip:*
Wear protective gloves during handling of the HAT medium— the aminopterin component is toxic.

Procedure:

1. On day 4 or 5 after fusion, aspirate 100 ml of old HAT medium (about half) from each well and replace with 2 drops of new HAT medium. Be careful not to disturb any cells which may be on the bottoms of the wells. After 7 to 10 days, you should screen the wells which have visible cell colonies or yellow supernatants for antibody production (see part E), and continue feeding only the antibody-positive wells as described below.

2. Continue feeding the hybridomas with HT medium for about 3 weeks. During this time, wells which have been screened as antibody-positive and have begun to turn the media yellow should be expanded to a larger culture. Remove the cells from a well by gently pipetting up and down with a micropipette. Transfer the cells from each well to a well in a 24-well culture plate with 0.5 mls HT medium. When the cells crowd the wells of the 24-well plate (the media will begin to turn yellow), transfer them to a 25cm^2 flask with 5 mls HT medium.

3. After 3 weeks, feed the cultures for 2 feedings with HT medium. Thereafter, the cultures may be maintained on regular growth medium with 10% serum, and split as necessary when the cultures become crowded.

E.   ELISA Screening for Antibody Production

The medium from each well can be assayed by ELISA for the presence of specific antibody anytime after the wells have visible cell colonies. This will occur anywhere from 7 to 10 days following fusion. Only the wells producing antibody of the desired specificity are selected for further culturing. Allow the cells to grow without feeding for 2-3 days prior to ELISA analysis. Use 50 μl of supernatant from each well to be tested, keeping track of every well.

Materials for Part E:

- ☐ 96-well microtiter plate with flat-bottomed wells
- ☐ 10 mls antigen solution (10 mg/ml in PBS)
- ☐ 10-ml pipettes
- ☐ phosphate buffered saline (PBS)
- ☐ blocking protein (1% gelatin in PBS)
- ☐ sample of known antibody against the antigen (control antiserum)
- ☐ 10 mls conjugate (rabbit anti-mouse IgG-Horse radish peroxidase)
- ☐ 10 mls substrate solution (5-aminosalicylic acid)
- ☐ 2 squirt bottles
- ☐ 200 µl automatic pipette and tips
- ☐ plastic wrap

Procedure:

1. *The following is to be done the day before or during the previous exercise.* Choose 4 wells on a 96-well, flat-bottom microtiter plate to designate as control wells (the first 4 wells of row A are most convenient). Label these wells 1A, 2A, 3A, 4A and 5A. Using a 10-ml pipette, add 2 drops of the antigen solution to control wells 2A, 3A, 4A and 5A. Do not add antigen to control well 1A. Also add two drops of antigen solution to enough wells for each hybridoma well you want to screen. Incubate the plate at 4°C until used.

2. Dump out the antigen solution by inverting the plate over the sink, then blotting dry on a stack of paper towels. *Completely* fill each well with blocking protein solution from a squirt bottle. Cover the plate with plastic wrap and incubate at 37°C for 15 minutes.

3. Wash the plate by filling the wells with PBS from a squirt bottle. Repeat once.

4. Add 50 µl of the supernatant from each hybridoma well to be tested to a well on the ELISA plate. Also add known anti-body to control wells 1A, 3A, 4A, and 5A. Incubate the plate for 30 minutes at 37°C.

5. Wash the plate two times with PBS as in step 3.

6. Add 50 µl of the conjugate to every well except control well 3A. Incubate for 30 minutes at 37°C.

7. Wash the plate three times in PBS as in step 3.

8. Add hydrogen peroxide to the substrate solution to a final concentration of 0.01%. Add 50 µl of the substrate solution to every well except control well 4A. Incubate for 15 to 30 minutes at 37°C. Positive wells will develop a brown color. Control wells 1A, 2A, 3A, and 4A should be negative. Control well 5A should be positive.

F.   Cloning By Limiting Dilution

Once the wells containing the desired hybridomas have been identified by ELISA and expanded to culture flasks, the cultures are diluted and plated so that one single cell is placed in one of the wells of a microtiter plate. These new wells are observed closely to make sure that only one clone (cell colony) is present in one of the wells. If more than one colony is found in a well, that well is eliminated from further manipulations. The isolated clone may now be expanded to a larger culture volume, and retested by ELISA to make sure it is producing antibody of the desired specificity. This antibody is now monoclonal antibody, and can be harvested from the culture fluid. Stock cultures of the clone can be stored frozen in aliquots. When needed, the frozen cells can be thawed and grown in bulk, or the cells can be injected into the peritoneal cavity of mice. Being transformed cells, they will cause a tumor in mice characterized by the production of large amounts of fluid called **ascites fluid**, which contains the monoclonal antibody and is exuded into the peritoneum where it can easily be harvested from the mouse.

Materials for Part F:

- ☐ 200 µl automatic pipette with sterile tips
- ☐ 10 mls hybridoma growth medium
- ☐ cell culture plates (96-well, flat-bottom)

Procedure:

1. Add 100 µl of hybridoma growth medium to each well of the microtiter plate.

2. Transfer 100 µl from a hybridoma culture to the top left well of the microtiter plate (well 1A). Mix well but gently by pipetting up and down three times.

3. Perform two-fold dilutions down the left-hand column of the plate (eight wells total), and discard 100 µl from the eighth well. Be sure to mix carefully between each dilution step, and discard the pipette tip when finished.

4. Perform two-fold dilutions across each row of the plate (12 wells per row). Mix between dilution steps and change tips between each row.

5. Incubate the plates at 37°C in 5 to 7% CO_2. Cell colonies should be visible after a few days. Identify all wells which have only one or two colonies under the microscope. After 7 to 10 days, these wells may be screened by ELISA and expanded.

Key Terms:

clone
polyclonal response
monoclonal antibody
myeloma cells
hybridoma cells
polyethylene glycol
hypoxanthine phosphoribosyl
  transferase
aminopterin
feeder cells
ELISA
ascites fluid

Questions:

1. How many different fusion products are formed and how is each eliminated to leave only hybridoma cells?

2. Why is Balb/c the mouse strain immunized to obtain spleen cells for this procedure?

3. What factors do the feeder cells supply to the hybridomas?

4. Why are the outer wells of the microtiter plate left empty?

5. How might monoclonal antibodies be used in cancer therapy?

Additional Reading:

1. Kohler, G., and C. Milstein. 1975. Continuous culture of fused cells secreting antibody of predefined specificity. Nature 256:495.

2. Milstein, C. 1980. Monoclonal antibodies. Sci. Am. 243(4):66

3. Yelton, D. E., and M. D. Scharff. 1981. Monoclonal antibodies: a powerful new tool in biology and medicine. Ann. Rev. Biochem. 50:657.

4. Harlow, E., and D. Lane. 1988. Antibodies: A Laboratory Manual. Cold Spring Harbor, New York: Cold Spring Harbor Laboratory.

5. Waldmann, T. A. 1991. Monoclonal antibodies in diagnosis and therapy. Science 252:1657.

22 Jerne Plaque Assay

Niels K. Jerne made several important contributions to Immunology. Jerne, along with Burnet, proposed the **clonal selection theory** of the antibody response in the 1950's. This theory states that lymphocytes capable of responding to all possible antigens are present even before contact with a specific antigen. Once an antigen is encountered, the appropriate B cell clone is "selected" for differentiation and proliferation. There is now much evidence which supports this theory, and the genetic-molecular basis for the enormous repertoire of antigen responses that are possible has begun to be understood.

Jerne also proposed the **idiotypic network theory**. The unique antigen-binding sites of antibody molecules ("idiotypic determinants") can them-selves be recognized by the body as immunogenic if enough of any one type accumulates. Thus, at the height of proliferation of a particular B cell clone during an immune response, new antibodies may be formed against the immune response antibodies, thereby controlling the magnitude of the response. It is thought that this may be one way the body has of preventing immune responses from "getting out of control."

The Jerne plaque assay, developed by Jerne and Nordin, is a method of detecting antibody-producing B cells from among a population of mixed lymphocytes. It is carried out by mixing spleen cells from a mouse that has been immunized against sheep erythrocytes with a suspension of the erythrocytes. The mixture of spleen cells and

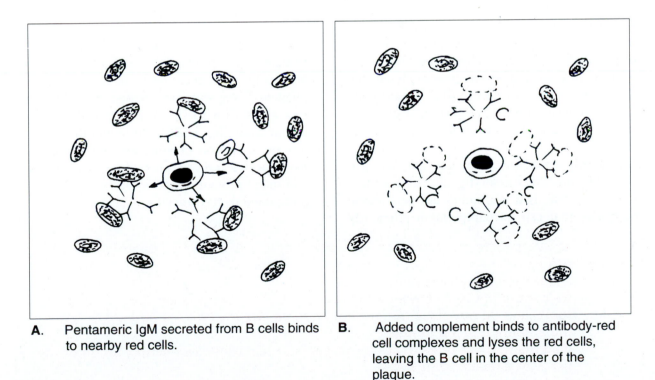

A. Pentameric IgM secreted from B cells binds to nearby red cells.

B. Added complement binds to antibody-red cell complexes and lyses the red cells, leaving the B cell in the center of the plaque.

Figure 22.1   Plaque formation in the Jerne Plaque Assay.

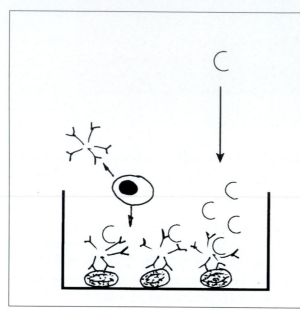

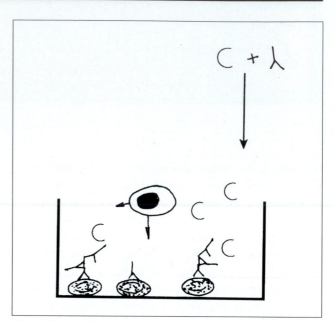

A. The direct assay. Complement is added to IgM-secreting B cells and red cells.

B. The indirect assay. Anti-IgG and complement are added to IgG-secreting B cells and red cells.

Figure 22.2   The Jerne Plaque Assay procedure.

erythrocytes is immobilized in agarose and incubated. Antibodies, being of molecular size, can easily diffuse through the agarose from the spleen B cells to bind to the the erythrocytes. If complement is then added to the agarose, it will join the bound antibody to lyse the erythrocytes. A clear plaque will form around each antibody-forming B cell as its neighboring erythrocytes are lysed (fig. 22.1). This assay is quantitative, because the number of plaque-forming cells (PFC) can be calculated by counting the plaques.

Only B cells which are producing IgM can form plaques by the direct assay (fig. 22.2A) described in this exercise. IgM antibodies are pentameric molecules that can fix complement efficiently

enough to form the plaques. Smaller antibodies like IgG require that two antibodies bind at adjacent sites on the erythrocyte membrane in order to fix complement. This is such a statistically rare event that plaques do not form directly with IgG. However, the Jerne plaque assay can be modified to detect cells producing other antibody classes besides IgM. For these tests, the number of complement fixing sites is increased by adding anti-IgG antiserum to the mixture in an indirect plaque assay (fig. 22.2B). Other modifications allow the detection of other antigen specificities. Erythrocytes from various species can be used, and many protein antigens can be used by coupling them to erythrocytes.

⚠ *Safety Tips:*
1.   **Avoid breathing anesthetic vapors.**
2.   **Be careful not to let ethanol drip down onto your hand when flaming dissection tools, and do not place hot dissection tools directly into the ethanol or touch the ethanol-doused mouse.**
3.   **If an ethanol fire does occur, don't panic or use water, but simply smother the fire with a beaker or towel.**
4.   **DEAE-dextran may be irritating to the skin. Wear gloves and avoid inhalation if handling the dry powder.**

Materials:

- ☐ two mice
- ☐ 2 1-ml syringes with 25-gauge needles
- ☐ 1 ml 20% washed sheep erythrocytes in phosphate buffered saline (PBS)
- ☐ 1 ml phosphate buffered saline (PBS)
- ☐ mouse jar, anesthetic, and cotton balls
- ☐ 70% ethanol in a squirt bottle
- ☐ dissecting tray, scissors, and forceps
- ☐ 95% ethanol in a jar
- ☐ 2 sterile petri plates each containing a piece of stainless steel mesh
- ☐ 2 15-ml centrifuge tubes
- ☐ 60 mls cold sterile cell culture medium (e.g. RPMI 1640)
- ☐ 5 sterile petri plates containing 20 mls of 1.4% agarose in cell culture medium, 2 or 3 days old
- ☐ 5 sterile tubes containing 2 mls of melted 0.7% agarose and 0.1% DEAE Dextran in cell culture medium, held at 45°C
- ☐ 10 mls of guinea pig complement, diluted 1:10 in PBS
- ☐ sterile 10-ml pipettes
- ☐ sterile 1-ml pipettes
- ☐ 45°C water bath
- ☐ 37°C water bath
- ☐ clinical centrifuge

Procedure:

1. Four days prior to this exercise, inject one mouse in the peritoneal cavity with 0.2 ml of the erythrocyte suspension. The injection technique should be demonstrated by your instructor (also see fig. 2.1). To inject the mouse, hold it at the base of the tail with your right hand (if you are right-handed), and let it cling to the top of its cage as you grasp the back of the neck with your left hand. You must pinch together all the loose skin right behind the ears between your thumb and the knuckle of your index finger so that the mouse is immobilized and cannot turn its head around to bite. Then lay the mouse across your hand with its back against your closed fingers, and clamp the tail and left leg of the mouse under your pinky. Insert the needle with the bevel facing up about 1/4 inch into the mouse's left lower abdomen and inject the suspension.

   The second mouse should be injected only with plain PBS as a control.

2. Let the agarose plates come to room temperature if they have been stored in a refrigerator. The soft agar tubes (0.7% agarose) should be melted and held in a 45°C water bath until needed.

3. Euthanize both mice by placing them in a jar or coffee can which contains a couple large cotton balls soaked in anesthetic. Close the jar tightly for 5 minutes.

4. For the remainder of the procedure, keep the spleens from each mouse, and the resulting cell suspensions, separate. Wet down a euthanized mouse with 70% ethanol. Sterilize a scissors and forceps by dipping them in 95% ethanol and passing them quickly through the Bunsen burner flame to burn off the alcohol. Pull up the skin of the abdomen with the sterile forceps and cut through the abdomen longitudinally with the scissors. Cut and fold back the skin of the abdomen to expose the internal organs.

5. Dip and flame the scissors and forceps again, then locate the spleen. The spleen is a long, flat, reddish organ lying directly under the stomach. Remove the spleen with the forceps (you may need to cut it free from connecting tissues) and place it in a sterile petri plate containing a screen (see fig. 21.3).

6. Add 10 mls of cell culture medium to the petri plate. Mince the spleen as finely as possible on the mesh using sterile (alcohol-flamed) scissors. Dip

the screen repeatedly into the wash medium to disperse the cells.

7. Transfer the spleen cell suspension into a 15-ml centrifuge tube. If large chunks of debris are present, let these settle for a few minutes, before transferring the suspension to the centrifuge tube. Discard the debris. Repeat steps 4–6 with the other mouse.

8. Centrifuge both spleen cell suspension at $500 \times g$ for 5 minutes. While the cells are spinning, pre-warm the complement solution in a 37°C water bath until needed.

9. After the centrifuge has come to a stop, remove the supernatant from the spleen cell pellets and discard. Resuspend each cell pellet in 10 mls cell culture medium. Hold the suspensions on ice.

10. Add 0.9 mls of cold cell culture medium to each of four small tubes, and label each tube "test," and with numbers 1–4. Prepare 10-fold dilutions of the spleen cell suspension from the immunized mouse by serially transferring 0.1 ml through each tube. Prepare another tube with 0.9 ml medium and label it "control." To this tube add 0.1 ml of the spleen cell suspension from the nonimmunized mouse. Hold all the tubes on ice.

11. Have the five melted soft agarose tubes ready in a water bath. Label four agarose plates "test." Also label each of these plates by the spleen cell dilution (i. e. "10^{-1}," "10^{-2}," "10^{-3}," or "10^{-4}") it will receive. Label the fifth plate "control."

12. Working quickly, add 0.1 ml of the erythrocyte suspension plus 0.1 ml of a "test" (immunized) spleen cell dilution to a tube of soft agarose. Mix by rolling the tube rapidly between your palms, then pour over the appropriate agarose

plate. Rock the plate as you pour to ensure even coverage by the soft agarose. Repeat this procedure with the remaining three "test" samples, then with the "control" sample.

13. Allow the top agarose layers to solidify completely (about 10 minutes), then incubate the plates in a 37°C incubator for 1 hour.

14. Flood each plate with 2 mls of the complement solution, then incubate for another 30 minutes at 37°C.

15. To look for plaques, view the plates under an inverted microscope or a dissecting microscope. A B-cell should be visible in the center of each plaque. Find a plate that has between 30 and 100 plaques on it. Count the plaques and calculate the #PFC/spleen, taking all dilution factors into account.

Key Terms:
clonal selection
idiotypic determinant

Questions:

1. How would you use the Jerne Plaque Assay to detect

   a) IgM-producing B cells?

   b) IgG-producing B cells?

   c) B cells producing IgM against a protein antigen?

2. In the Jerne Plaque Assay, why are mice immunized four days prior to the experiment?

Additional Reading:

1. Jerne, N. K., A. A. Nordin, and C. Henry. 1963. The Agar Plaque Technique for Recognizing Antibody-Producing Cells. Pp. 109–125 *in* Cell-Bound Antibodies. B. Amos and H. Koprowski, eds. Philadelphia, Pennsylvania: Wistar Institute Press.

2. Jerne, N. K., et al. 1974. Plaque forming cells: methodology and theory. Transplantation Reviews 18:130-191.

23 Lymphocyte Proliferation Assay

The cell mediated **immune response** can be evaluated by many methods. One simple method is skin testing for **delayed-type hypersensitivity** (DTH) reactions (e.g. allergy testing or the Mantoux test for tuberculosis). However, skin tests are not always reliable. The **lymphocyte proliferation assay** is a more useful and versatile test which relies on the use of lectins.

Lectins are substances of plant or bacterial origin which have the ability to stimulate cellular mitosis. They are also called mitogens. Some commonly used lectins include **phytohemagglutinin** (PHA) which stimulates mature T cells to divide, **concanavalin A** (ConA), which is mitogenic for both mature and immature T-cells, and **pokeweed mitogen** (PWM), which stimulates both T and B-cells.

Mitogen-stimulated lymphocytes exhibit an increase in their rate of protein and nucleic acid synthesis. This increase in growth can be measured by adding **tritiated thymidine**, a radioisotope-labeled DNA precursor, to the cell culture medium. The amount of tritium taken up by the cultured cells following mitogen exposure is correlated to the level of cellular proliferation.

Mitogen-induced lymphocyte proliferation is used by researchers and clinicians to distinguish T and B cells and identify a variety of deficiencies in the immune response. Some variations of this type of assay include the **mixed lymphocyte response** (MLR), and the **cell mediated lympholysis reaction** (CTL). In the MLR, populations of allogeneic lymphocytes are mixed together, and their proliferative response to each other's Major Histocompatibility Complex (MHC) class II antigens is measured by tritiated thymidine uptake. In the CTL reaction, the response of lymphocytes to the MHC class I antigens of foreign target cells is quantified by release of a radioactive label from the target cells upon lysis by T cytotoxic (Tc) cells. Both assays are useful in tissue matching for transplantation.

For this exercise, you will perform the lymphocyte proliferation assay on spleen cells of the mouse.

> ⚠ **WARNING:**
> **This exercise uses several hazardous reagents. Read all the safety information carefully before starting (including appendix 5C).**

A. Preparation of Mouse spleen cells

Materials for Parts A and B:
- [ ] mouse
- [ ] mouse jar, anesthetic, and cotton balls
- [ ] 70% ethanol in a squirt bottle
- [ ] dissecting tray, scissors, and forceps
- [ ] 95% ethanol in a jar
- [ ] sterile petri plate containing a piece of stainless steel mesh
- [ ] 50 mls wash medium (RPMI without serum)
- [ ] 20 mls growth medium (RPMI containing 10% fetal bovine serum, 2-mercaptoethanol (5×10^{-5} M), gentamicin (50 µg/ml) or penicillin (100 U/ml)/streptomycin (100 µg/ml)
- [ ] 15-ml sterile centrifuge tube
- [ ] small glass tube
- [ ] hemocytometer and trypan blue dye
- [ ] sterile 1-ml cotton-plugged pipettes
- [ ] sterile 10-ml cotton-plugged pipettes
- [ ] sterile Pasteur pipettes and bulb
- [ ] clinical centrifuge

139

Procedure:

1.   Euthanize a mouse by placing it in a jar or coffee can which contains a large cotton ball soaked in anesthetic. Close the jar tightly for 5 minutes.

2.   Use careful aseptic technique for the following procedures. Wet down the euthanized mouse with 70% ethanol. Sterilize a scissors and forceps by dipping them in 95% ethanol and passing them quickly through the Bunsen burner flame to burn off the alcohol. Pull up the skin of the abdomen with the sterile forceps and cut through the abdomen longitudinally with the scissors. Cut and fold back the skin of the abdomen to expose the internal organs.

3.   Dip and flame the scissors and forceps again, then locate the spleen. The spleen is a long, flat, reddish organ lying directly under the stomach. Remove the spleen with the forceps (you may need to cut it free from connecting tissues) and place it in the sterile petri plate containing the steel mesh (see fig. 21.3).

4.   Add 10 ml of wash medium to the petri plate. Mince the spleen as finely as possible on the mesh using sterile (alcohol-flamed) scissors. Dip the mesh repeatedly into the wash medium to disperse the cells.

5.   Transfer the spleen cell suspension to a 15-ml centrifuge tube. Set aside 0.5 ml in a small tube for counting the cells.

6.   Centrifuge the spleen cell suspension at $200 \times g$ for 5 minutes. Meanwhile, count the cells you set aside using a hemocytometer and trypan blue stain (see part B). Calculate the volume of medium needed to resuspend the cell pellet to a concentration of 5×10^6 viable cells/ml.

7.   After the centrifuge has come to a stop, discard the supernatant and gently resuspend the cell pellet in 10 mls wash medium by pipetting up and down ten times. Repeat centrifugation at $200 \times g$ for 5 minutes.

8.   Wash cells once more as in step 7.

9.   Discard the supernatant and resuspend the cell pellet in the appropriate volume of *growth* medium as calculated in step 6.

B.   Counting Cells With a Hemocytometer

Procedure:

1.   Mix a small amount of the cell suspension with an equal volume of trypan blue solution. Mix thoroughly by pipetting up and down with a Pasteur pipette, and allow to stand for 10 minutes.

2.   Meanwhile, clean the hemocytometer and coverslip with 70% ethanol and lens paper.

3.   With the coverslip in place on the hemocytometer, use a Pasteur pipette to

transfer the cell suspension/dye mixture to both chambers. Carefully touch the edge of the chamber to the pipette tip and allow the chamber to fill by capillary action. Do not overfill or underfill the chambers.

4. Starting with one chamber, count all the cells in the four 1 mm corner squares (see figure 23.1). Keep a separate count of the number of viable cells and dead cells (dead cells stain blue). For cells lying on a line, count those which lie on top or left lines of the squares, but not those which lie on bottom or right lines of the squares.

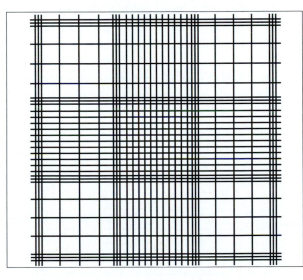

Figure 23.1   Hemocytometer Grid

5. Count the second chamber in the same manner as the first.

6. The hemocytometer chamber represents a volume of 0.1 mm^3, or 1×10^{-4} cm^3. Because 1 cm^3 is equivalent to 1 ml, the cell concentration per ml can be calculated using a chamber volume conversion factor of 10^4 in the following equation:

$$\# \ cells/ml = \ average \ count/square$$
$$\times \ dilution factor$$
$$\times \ chamber \ conversion \ factor$$

e.g., if 200 cells were counted in one chamber from a 1:2 dilution of cells in trypan blue, the number of cells per ml in the original suspension is calculated as:

$$\frac{200 \ cells \ counted}{4 \ squares} \times 2 \times 10^4 = 1 \times 10^6 \ cells/ml$$

The total number of cells in the original sample is then:

$$\# \ cells/ml \times total \ volume \ of \ sample \ (ml)$$

Which, for a 10 ml suspension would be:

$$1 \times 10^6 \ cells/ml \times 10 \ ml = 1 \times 10^7 \ total \ cells$$

7. If the cells appear clustered or there is more than 10% variation in the cell counts between chambers, repeat the count after dispersing the cells in the original suspension and then the dye dilution by vigorous pipetting.

8. If there are less than 100 or greater than 400 cells to count (25–100 cells per 1 mm square), repeat the procedure after adjusting the cells to an appropriate dilution (this dilution factor must be taken into account in the calculations).

9. There should not be less than 95% viability of the cells.

C.   Preparation of Assay Plate

Materials for Part C:
- ☐ 20 mls growth medium
- ☐ mitogens: PHA (200 µg/ml), ConA (200 µg/ml), and PWM (200 µg/ml)
- ☐ cell culture plate (96-well, round-bottom)
- ☐ sterile 10-ml cotton-plugged pipettes
- ☐ 200 µl and 1000 µl automatic pipettes with sterile tips
- ☐ 24 sterile test tubes
- ☐ 37°C incubator

⚠️ **Safety Tip:**

Wear doubled protective gloves when handling the mitogens. PHA and ConA are possible teratogens and are very toxic, especially in concentrated form. Handle only the diluted working solutions. PWM is an irritant and may cause sensitization by skin contact.

Procedure:

1. Prepare a rack containing 3 rows of test tubes, 8 tubes per row. Label the rows A (PHA), B (ConA), and C (PWM).

2. Add 0.5 ml growth medium to each tube using a 10-ml pipette.

3. Using a 1000 µl automatic pipette, prepare two-fold dilutions of each mitogen by transferring 0.5 ml (500 µl) volumes through the 8 tubes in each row. Be sure to use new tips for each transfer. You should now have concentrations ranging from approximately 100 to 0.8 µg/ml for each mitogen.

4. Using a 200 µl automatic pipette, add 0.1 ml of each mitogen dilution to each of 3 wells in the microtiter plate according to the pattern shown in figure 23.2— that is, each dilution in triplicate.

5. Place 0.1 ml of plain growth medium in 3 additional wells to serve as negative controls.

6. Add 0.1 ml of the spleen cell suspension to each mitogen and control well.

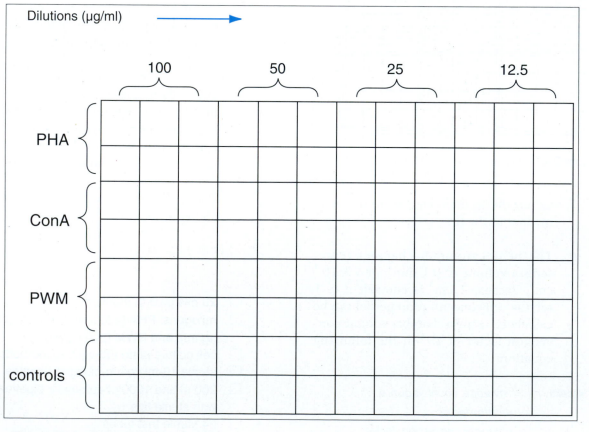

Figure 23.2   Pattern for assay plate.

7. Place the microtiter plate in a CO_2 incubator at 37°C for 48 hours.

D.   Radioisotope Labeling ("Pulse")

Because mitosis involves the production of new DNA, cell proliferation is correlated to the amount of DNA synthesized. This can be quantified by measuring the cellular uptake of ^{3}H-thymidine from the culture medium. The amount of radioactivity taken up is measured after a short exposure to the labeled precursor following mitogen treatment.

⚠️ *Safety Tip:*

Special procedures must be employed when working with radioactive materials. The proper precautions must be thoroughly discussed by the instructor before beginning work.

Materials for Part D:
- ☐ ^{3}H-thymidine solution (50 μCi in 2 mls)
- ☐ repeating dispenser (20 μl delivery)
- ☐ gloves
- ☐ plastic tray and absorbent pad
- ☐ 37°C incubator

Procedure:

1. Using a repeating dispenser (instructor will demonstrate its use), add 20 μl of the ^{3}H-thymidine solution to each well. This will result in the delivery of 0.5 μCi per well.

2. Incubate the culture plate in a tray placed in the incubator. Incubate at 37°C in 5% CO_2 for 24 hours.

E.   Cell Harvesting and Measurement of ^{3}H-thymidine Uptake

Tritium (^{3}H) emits β-radiation. Beta radiation is low energy atomic decay due to the release of particles from the nucleus. Because the radiation is low energy it is difficult to detect. Therefore, a liquid scintillant ("cocktail") is usually used to convert β-particles into photons of light which can be measured spectrophotometrically in a scintillation counter. The scintillant usually consists of fluorochrome compounds dissolved in toluene.

Toluene absorbs the energy from the β-particle and passes off an electron to the fluorochrome, which then releases the energy as a photon of light (figure 23.3). The toluene is incompatible with aqueous or polar samples and can only be used if the sample is completely dried onto a filter paper.

Materials:
- ☐ Assay plate
- ☐ cell harvester apparatus
- ☐ glass fiber filter paper
- ☐ absorbent pad
- ☐ gloves
- ☐ forceps
- ☐ 75 7-ml plastic mini-vials for scintillation
- ☐ 200 mls scintillation cocktail

Procedure:

1. After the 24-hour pulse, harvest the cells in each well onto filter paper with a cell harvester. This is an instrument which will draw the materials from the well onto the paper and wash it. The instructor will demonstrate its use.

2. Place the filter paper strip containing the samples in a 37°C incubator for 60 minutes. Make sure to lay the strip on the disposable pad. Meanwhile, label 75 vial caps with the sample number and your initials.

3. After drying, place the filter paper disc obtained from each well in a vial. Add 2 mls cocktail and close with a labeled cap. Make sure the paper disc is submerged in the cocktail.

4. Load the vials in the scintillation counter and program to count each vial for 1 minute.

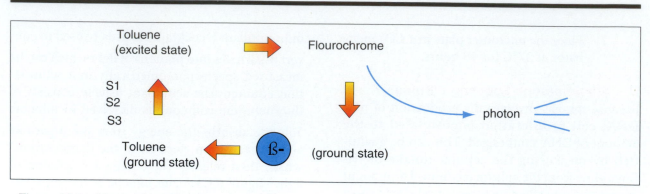

Figure 23.3   Mechanism of action of scintillant.

⚠ **Safety Tip:**

The scintillation cocktail contains a volatile solvent. It should be dispensed in a fume hood. Radiation safety practices must continue.

F.   Results

The measurements from the counter will be presented as **counts per minute** (cpms). The control and test dilutions were performed in triplicate, so each set of 3 cpms must be averaged together and expressed as the mean cpms for the dilution. Record the results in table 23.1. The standard error should be calculated for each mean. Variations in the cpms of individual wells that vary by more than 20% of the mean are due to error, and these wells should be eliminated from the re-calculation.

Error may be due to omission of the tritium pulse to that well or cell death due to contamination (resulting in cpms which are too low), or bacterial growth (resulting in cpms which are too high).

When the mean cpms have been calculated, plot the cpms versus mitogen concentration for each mitogen on linear graph paper.

Key Terms:
CMI
skin testing
delayed-type hypersensitivity
lymphocyte proliferation assay
lectin
mitogen
tritiated thymidine
scintillation cocktail
scintillation counter
counts per minute
β radiation

Table 23.1   Results of ^{3}H-thymidine Count

Mitogen (µg/ml) concentration	cpms PHA	cpms ConA	cpms PWM
100			
50			
25			
12.5			
6.25			
3.13			
1.5			
0.75			

Questions:

1. What relative proportions of B-cells and T-cells were found in the spleen?

2. What proportions would you expect if the thymus were the organ used?

3. What is the purpose of the 2-mercaptoethanol in the growth medium? The antibiotics?

4. Why does bacterial growth in the wells cause an increased cpm?

5. What is the similarity between a mitogen and an antigen? What is the difference?

6. Should there be any difference between PHA and ConA stimulation in spleen cells? Why or Why not?

7. What was the optimal concentration of each mitogen for lymphocyte stimulation?

Additional Reading:

1. Mishell, B. B., and S. M. Shiigi. 1980. Selected Methods in Cellular Immunology. San Francisco: W. H. Freeman and Co.

2. Nowell, P. C. 1960. PHA: an initiator of mitosis in cultures of normal human leukocytes. Cancer Res. 20:562.

3. Pick, A. B., and F. H. Bach. 1973. A miniaturized mouse mixed lymphocyte culture in serum-free and mouse serum supplemented media. J. Immunol. Meth. 3:147.

24   Mixed Lymphocyte Response

In the previous exercise, the proliferation of lymphocytes in response to several mitogenic substances was measured. Lymphocytes will also proliferate in response to antigens. For most antigens, prior exposure to the antigen is required in order to elicit a response that is measurable by the proliferation assay. However, certain surface antigens of cells induce proliferation in the assay without prior exposure to the antigens. These surface antigens are called **major histocompatibility complex** (MHC) antigens. Because the MHC antigens differ between individuals, they are **allogeneic** antigens and are one of the major causes of organ rejection following transplantation. It is these antigens that must be carefully matched in the search for an organ donor.

All nucleated cells possess class I MHC antigens. Immune cells possess additional class II MHC antigens which also function in "self" recognition in the immune response. If lymphocytes from two different individuals are mixed together, they will proliferate in response to each other's MHC antigens. This response can be measured in an assay known as the **Mixed Lymphocyte Response** (MLR). In this exercise you will carry out an MLR assay using spleen cells from two different strains of mice (allogeneic individuals). You will also carry out a second MLR using spleen cells from two mice of the same strain (syngeneic individuals). Because mice within the same strain are genetically identical, these cells should show no greater level of proliferation than would be expected from normal cell growth. The MLR assay is set up in much the same way as the lymphocyte proliferation assay.

Materials:
- ☐ 2 mice of the same strain (e.g. Balb/c)
- ☐ 1 mouse of a different strain (e.g. C57BL6)
- ☐ mouse jar, anesthetic, and cotton balls
- ☐ 70% ethanol in squirt bottle
- ☐ dissecting tray, scissors, and forceps
- ☐ 95% ethanol in a jar
- ☐ sterile petri plate containing a piece of stainless steel mesh
- ☐ 50 mls wash medium (RPMI without serum)
- ☐ 20 mls growth medium (RPMI containing 10% fetal bovine serum, 2-mercaptoethanol (5×10^{-5} M), gentamicin (50 µg/ml) or penicillin (100 U/ml)/streptomycin (100 µg/ml)
- ☐ cell culture plate (96-well, round-bottom)
- ☐ 15-ml sterile centrifuge tube
- ☐ small glass tube
- ☐ hemocytometer and trypan blue dye
- ☐ sterile 1-ml cotton-plugged pipettes
- ☐ sterile 10-ml cotton-plugged pipettes
- ☐ sterile Pasteur pipettes and bulb
- ☐ 37°C incubator

⚠ **Safety Tips:**
1. **Special procedures must be employed when working with radioactive materials. The proper precautions must be thoroughly discussed by the instructor before beginning work.**
2. **The scintillation cocktail contains a volatile solvent. It should be dispensed in a fume hood.**
3. **Avoid breathing anesthetic vapors.**

Procedure:

1. Euthanize the three mice and remove the spleens (keep all three spleens and the resulting cell suspensions separate from each other). Prepare cell suspensions from the three cells and wash the cells in exactly the same manner as in exercise 23, part A. The final suspensions should be at a concentration of 5×10^6 cells/ml in growth medium.

2. To three wells in the first row of the assay plate, add 0.1 ml cell suspension from each of two different mouse strains. Each well in this first row will then contain a 0.2-ml mixture of allogeneic cells.

3. To three wells in the second row of the assay plate, add 0.1 ml cell suspension from each of the two identical mouse strains. Each well in this row will contain a 0.2-ml mixture of nonresponding cells.

4. To three wells of the third row of the assay plate, add 0.2 mls of cell suspension from one mouse (either strain will do). This row is a control which will show the amount of cell proliferation to be expected from normal cell growth.

5. Incubate the assay plate at 37°C in a 5% CO_2 incubator for 4 days.

6. After 4 days, pulse each well with 0.5 μCi ^{3}H-thymidine as in exercise 23, part D. Harvest the cells 24 hours later as in exercise 23, part E. Calculate average cpms for wells within the same row, and compare the proliferation of the allogeneic cells to the nonresponding cells. Record your results in table 24.1.

Table 24.1 Results

cell types	average cpms
allogeneic	
syngeneic	
control cells	

Key Terms:

major histocompatibility antigens
allogeneic
syngeneic
mixed lymphocyte response

Questions:

1. How might you modify this experiment in order to measure the proliferative response of only one population of cells to the other cell type?

Additional Reading:

1. Mishell, B. B., and S. M. Shiigi. 1980. Selected Methods in Cellular Immunology. San Francisco: W. H. Freeman and Co.

2. Bach, F., and K. Hirschorn. 1964. Lymphocyte interaction: a potential histocompatibility test in vitro. Science 143:813.

3. Pick, A. B., and F. H. Bach. 1973. A miniaturized mouse mixed lymphocyte culture in serum-free and mouse serum supplemented media. J. Immunol. Methods 3:147.

25 Antibody-Mediated Cytolysis

Progress in understanding how the cells of the immune system interact during the immune response is due in part to the ability to separate and identify the various subpopulations of lymphocytes. In an earlier exercise, a simple method for identifying T-cell lymphocytes by rosetting was demonstrated. because the T-cells are themselves divided into several subpopulations, a means of identifying T-cell types is necessary in order to define the functions of these cells.

Each subset of T-cells has unique surface antigens, as well as antigens that are shared by all thymocyte-derived cells. By treatment of T-cells with serum complement plus antibody directed against any one of these specific or shared antigens, functional subpopulations of cells can be depleted from a mixture. Cells are opsonized by specific antibody, then killed by the complement proteins. Damage to the cell membrane is evidenced by the uptake of trypan blue or nigrosin dyes. By using different combinations of the antibodies, all cells in a mixture except the cell type of interest can be removed, leaving a single, isolated cell type viable for further study. This technique is called antibody-mediated cytolysis, and is used along with the MLR assay (exercise 24) in tissue typing for transplantation, as well as in research studies of cell function.

In this exercise, you will use antibody-mediated cytolysis to determine the proportions of different T-cell types in the mouse spleen and thymus (see Table 25.1). The murine Thy-1 antigen is present on all T cells, and in this way is analogous to the human CD3 or CD2 (rosette-binding receptor) antigens. The murine Ly2 antigen is associated with MHC class I restricted activities and occurs on cytotoxic and suppressor T cells. It is analogous to the human CD8 population of T cells. The murine L3T4 antigen is a marker for MHC class II restricted activities and occurs on T helper and T delayed-type hypersensitivity cells. It is analogous to the human CD4 T cell antigen. There are many more lymphocyte markers in addition to those presented here.

Materials:

- ☐ mouse
- ☐ mouse jar, anesthetic, and cotton balls
- ☐ squirt bottle containing 70% ethanol
- ☐ jar containing 95% ethanol
- ☐ dissecting tray, scissors, and forceps
- ☐ 2 sterile petri plates, one containing a piece of stainless steel mesh
- ☐ wash medium (RPMI 1640 medium (without BSA))
- ☐ assay medium (RPMI 1640 medium with 0.3% bovine serum albumin (BSA))
- ☐ 4 15-ml centrifuge tubes
- ☐ glass test tubes
- ☐ 1 ml T-cell antigen-specific antibody
- ☐ 2 mls low toxicity rabbit complement
- ☐ 1-ml pipettes
- ☐ Pasteur pipettes and bulb
- ☐ 0.2% nigrosin dye in saline
- ☐ hemocytometer
- ☐ ice bucket
- ☐ 37°C water bath
- ☐ clinical centrifuge

⚠ **Safety Tips:**
1. **Avoid breathing anesthetic vapors.**
2. **Be careful not to let ethanol drip down onto your hand when flaming dissection tools, and do not place hot dissection tools directly into the ethanol or touch the ethanol-doused mouse.**
3. **If an ethanol fire does occur, don't panic or use water, but simply smother the fire with a beaker or towel.**

Procedure:

1. Euthanize a mouse by placing it in a jar or coffee can which contains a large cotton ball soaked in anesthetic. Close the jar tightly for 5 minutes.

2. Use careful aseptic technique for the following procedures. Wet down the euthanized mouse with 70% ethanol. Sterilize a scissors and forceps by dipping them in 95% ethanol and passing them quickly through the Bunsen burner flame to burn off the alcohol. Pull up the skin of the abdomen with the sterile forceps and cut through the abdomen longitudinally with the scissors. Cut and fold back the skin of the abdomen to expose the internal organs.

3. Dip and flame the scissors and forceps again, then locate either the spleen or the thymus. The spleen is a long, flat, reddish organ lying directly under the stomach. The thymus is the grayish organ lying directly on top of the heart. Remove either the spleen or thymus with the forceps (you may need to cut it free from connecting tissues) and place the organ in a sterile petri plate.

4. Add 10 ml of wash medium to the petri plate, then transfer the organ to a second petri plate. Add 10 mls wash media to the plate and mince the organ as finely as possible on a screen using sterile (alcohol-flamed) scissors. Dip the screen repeatedly into the wash medium to disperse the cells.

5. Transfer the cell suspension to a 15-ml centrifuge tube. Set aside 0.5 ml in a small tube for counting the cells.

6. Centrifuge the cell suspension at 200 × g for 5 minutes. Meanwhile, count the cells you set aside using a hemocytometer and trypan blue stain (see exercise 23, part B). Calculate the volume of medium needed to resuspend the cell pellet to a concentration of 5×10^6 **viable** cells/ml.

7. After the centrifuge has come to a stop, discard the supernatant and gently resuspend the cell pellet in 10 mls wash medium by pipetting up and down ten times. Repeat centrifugation at 200 × g for 5 minutes.

8. Discard the supernatant and resuspend the cell pellet in the appropriate volume of **growth** medium as calculated in step 6.

9. Add 1 ml of the cell suspension to each of three new 15-ml centrifuge tubes which have been labeled as follows:

   'A'—untreated control
   'B'—complement control
   'C'—antibody + complement

If you are testing more than one antigen, label additional antibody + complement tubes, along with the name of the antigen being tested.

10. Centrifuge the tubes at 200 × g for 5 minutes to pellet the cells. Discard the supernatants and resuspend the pellets as follows:

    'A'—1 ml RPMI + 0.3% BSA
    'B'—1 ml RPMI + 0.3% BSA
    'C'—1 ml T cell antigen-specific
        antiserum

11. Incubate all tubes in a 4°C ice bath for 30 minutes.

12. Centrifuge the tubes again to pellet the cells at 200 × g for 5 minutes. Discard the supernatants and resuspend the pellets as follows:

    'A'—1 ml RPMI + 0.3% BSA
    'B'—1 ml complement
    'C'—1 ml complement

13. Incubate all tubes in a 37°C water bath for 30 minutes.

14. Place the tubes on ice. Dilute each sample 1:10 in 0.2% nigrosin dye and let sit 10 minutes.

15. Count 100 cells on the hemocytometer from each sample. Record how many cells from the 100 are dead and how many are viable. Determine the percent cell death for each sample.

16. The control samples should have less than 5% cell death. Determine the percentage of cells in sample 'C' which carry the specific antigen.

Table 25.1   Proportion of Cells Expressing Thy-1, L3T4 and Ly2 Antigens in the Mouse Spleen and Thymus

Organ	Thy-1	Antigen L3T4 (CD4)	Ly2 (CD8)
Spleen	35	24	11
Thymus	>98	90	85

Questions:

1. Describe two techniques which can help eliminate graft rejection.

Additional Reading:

1. Mishell, B. B., and S. M. Shiigi. 1980. Selected Methods in Cellular Immunology. San Francisco: W. H. Freeman and Co.

2. Coligan, J. E. et al., eds. 1991. Current Protocols in Immunology. New York: Greene Publishing Associates and Wiley-Interscience.

26 Ammonium Sulfate Precipitation of Antibody

The serum proteins constitute about 6% of normal serum, and are classified as either albumins or globulins. The globulins consist of the alpha, beta, and gamma groups. Antibodies, which make up about 10% of the total protein, are globulins that occur in the beta and gamma groups. It is desirable for many procedures to have a more concentrated and pure sample of antibody than that offered by an antiserum. The serum proteins exhibit significant differences in their solubilities based on their net charges at a given pH. Normally, proteins are soluble in water because their exposed polar groups form hydrogen bonds with water molecules. However, if high concentrations of small, highly charged ions are added to the solution, the small ions will compete with the proteins for binding with water. The ions have the effect of removing the water from the protein, thereby reducing the solubility of the protein and causing it to precipitate out of solution. How much the solubility of each individual protein is reduced by the addition of the ions depends on the ion concentration and the net charge of the particular protein at a given pH. Certain salt solutions such as 50% $(NH_4)_2SO_4$ or 18% Na_2SO_4 will selectively precipitate globulins out of serum, leaving the albumins soluble in the supernatant. The crude globulin precipitate can then be collected by centrifugation and resolubilized, but will contain a mixture of alpha, beta, and gamma globulins, as well as a small amount of contaminating albumin trapped within the precipitate lattice. Steps can be taken to further purify the antibody fraction of the globulin preparation if necessary.

For this exercise, you will perform an ammonium sulfate "salt cut" of an antiserum (part A). The globulin you isolate will be further purified by immunoaffinity techniques in the next exercise. Because the globulin precipitate will contain ammonium ions that could interfere with later procedures, you will also "de-salt" the globulin by equilibrium dialysis (part B).

A. Precipitation

Materials:
- ☐ 3 mls heterogeneous antiserum
- ☐ 3 mls of a saturated solution of $(NH_4)_2SO_4$ (76 g/100 ml)
- ☐ 2N NaOH and HCl in dropper bottles
- ☐ 2 mls phosphate buffered saline (PBS)
- ☐ 50-ml centrifuge tube
- ☐ glass stir rod
- ☐ ice bucket
- ☐ dialysis tubing (12,000-14,000 MW)
- ☐ 2 tubing clamps (labeled with the same number)
- ☐ Pasteur pipette and bulb
- ☐ clinical centrifuge

Procedure:

1. Obtain 2 or 3 mls of antiserum. Centrifuge the antiserum at 1800 × g for 30 minutes to clarify. Discard any pelleted debris that is present after centrifugation.

2. Transfer the antiserum to a 15-ml centrifuge tube, reserving 0.5 mls in a small freezer tube for use in the PAGE in exercise 28. Place the centrifuge tube in an ice bucket to chill.

3. Adjust the pH of the saturated ammonium sulfate before use to pH 7.8 by adding drops of HCl or NaOH and testing with litmus paper. Place on ice to chill.

4.   After the antiserum has chilled (5 to 10 minutes), add slowly (drop-wise) with constant stirring, an equal volume of chilled ammonium sulfate. A white precipitate should form.

5.   Leave the tube at 0 to 4°C overnight.

6.   Following overnight incubation, centrifuge the precipitated antiserum at 1800 × g for 30 minutes.

7.   Discard the supernatant, and drain the tube well. Dissolve the precipitate in a volume of PBS equal to half the starting volume of the antiserum.

8.   The globulin fraction is now ready for desalting by dialysis, as follows.

B.   Dialysis of Antibody Solution

After preparing the globulin fraction of the serum, it will be necessary to remove the ammonium ions. To do this, you will use a dialysis method, although gel filtration could also be used. Dialysis tubing is a semipermeable nitrocellulose membrane which allows the separation of molecules by diffusion. The tubing is manufactured in various pore-size ranges. because immunoglobulins are large molecular weight proteins, it is easy to separate them from the salt ions by using tubing of pore-size 12,000 to 14,000 molecular weight. When the dialysis tubing is filled with the sample and placed into a buffer solution, the small salt molecules will pass through the pores and into the buffer by diffusion, while the proteins will remain trapped inside. Salt will stop diffusing from inside the tubing when its concentration reaches equilibrium on both sides of the membrane. By changing the buffer solution several times, most of the salt can be removed from the sample.

Materials for Part B:

☐ dialysis tubing (12,000–14,000 exclusion limit) and tubing clamps
☐ large beaker
☐ 2-liter Erlenmeyer flask
☐ magnetic stir plate and stir bar
☐ 8 liters phosphate buffered saline (PBS)
☐ 15-ml centrifuge tube
☐ Pasteur pipettes and bulb
☐ clinical centrifuge

Procedure:

1.   Cut an approximately 12-inch length of dialysis tubing. Soak it in a beaker of distilled water about 10 minutes, then rinse it in 3 changes of distilled water. Do not allow the tubing to dry once it has been soaked.

2.   Clamp one end of the tubing shut, being careful not to stretch the tubing and possibly enlarge the pores. Using a Pasteur pipette, place the antibody into the tubing, leaving an equal volume of space to allow for expansion. Clamp the top shut.

3.   Place the filled tubing in a large flask containing 2 liters of PBS and a magnetic stir bar (see fig. 7.2). Stir gently at 4°C.

4.   Change the PBS three times over a period of 1 to 2 days.

5.   After the dialysis is complete, carefully unclamp one end of the tubing and transfer the antibody to a 15-ml tube. If there is debris or precipitate present in the solution, centrifuge at 1800 × g for 15 minutes and transfer the globulin to a new tube. Discard the debris.

Additional Reading:

1. Mishell, B. B., and S. M. Shiigi. 1980. Selected Methods in Cellular Immunology. San Francisco: W. H. Freeman and Co.

2. Coligan, J. E., et al., eds. 1991. Current Protocols in Immunology. New York: Greene Publishing Associates and Wiley-Interscience.

27 Affinity Chromatography

Affinity chromatography is a simple and effective method of purifying biological substances. The term was coined in 1968 by Cuatrecasas, et al., although the basic concept was first described by Starkenstein in 1910 and was used to purify antibody by Campbell in 1951.

The technique involves treating an insoluble support matrix such as agarose beads with chemicals which make the support material reactive to binding a **ligand**. The ligand can be virtually any molecule which has an active chemical group available for covalent binding to the support, and the ability to bind specifically but reversibly to the molecule to be purified. By passing the mixture containing the molecule to be purified over a column of the matrix with its bound ligand, the molecule of interest will bind to the ligand while the other molecules in the mixture can be washed through the column. The purified molecule can then be released from the column (usually by changing the pH of the buffer) because its binding is reversible. Antibodies can be used as ligands to purify an antigen, and antigens can be used as ligands to purify specific antibody. Other types of biochemical interactions can also be exploited, such as hormones and their receptors, or enzymes and substrates.

Today, supports having almost any property desired can be developed, and by taking advantage of biospecific or immunological interactions of the ligand, virtually any protein or other macromolecule can be purified on the ligand-bound support. The technique is the most frequently used method of purifying antigen-specific antibody from a sample of polyclonal antiserum.

For this exercise, either of two "batch" purification procedures may be utilized. In part 1, a **protein A** ligand is used to purify IgG antibody from the crude globulin salt cut prepared in the pre-vious exercise. Protein A is a 42,000-dalton polypeptide derived from the cell wall of the bacterium *Staphylococcus aureus*. It has a high affinity for the Fc portion of antibody molecules from several animal species, including rabbits and humans (see figure 27.1). Several similar proteins, such as protein G from *Streptococcus*, have also been found. Although no biological explanation for the high affinity of these proteins for antibody has ever been discovered, they have become very useful reagents in affinity purification, ELISA testing, and other immunological procedures.

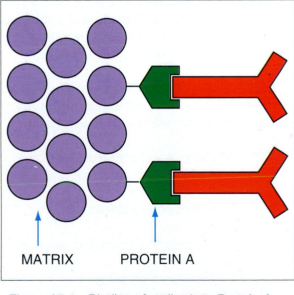

Figure 27.1   Binding of antibody to Protein-A matrix.

In part 2, a carbonyldiimidazole-activated (CDI) agarose gel is used to bind the ligand. This type of activated gel matrix can be used to bind almost any protein ligand. In this exercise, the ligand is the specific antigen which is recognized by the antibodies you are purifying. Preparation of this type of gel requires several more steps because you will have to bind the ligand to the gel by yourself, but the advantage is that you can purify antibody of a single antigen specificity. With protein A gels, all antibodies present in a serum sample are purified together, regardless of antigen specificity.

Treatment with CDI makes the agarose beads in the gel matrix reactive to proteins. Proteins are covalently bound to the gel beads by the chemical reaction shown in figure 27.2. It is necessary to make sure the particular protein antigen you are using is bound efficiently by the activated gel, because the amount of binding can vary between different proteins. Therefore, after the protein has been allowed to react with the gel for two days, you will measure the amount of protein left unbound in the gel supernatant using the Bio-Rad™ assay.

Once the antigen ligand is bound to the gel, antiserum can be passed through the gel just as with the protein A gel, and specific antibodies will bind the immobilized ligand. The purified antibodies can then be released from the gel by altering the pH of the buffer that is run through the gel.

Polyacrylamide gel electrophoresis will be carried out in the next exercise to determine the purity of the IgG obtained by affinity chromatography.

Part 1:   Protein A Affinity Purification

Materials for Part 1:
- ☐ Pasteur pipettes and bulb
- ☐ glass stir rod
- ☐ salt-cut globulin fraction from exercise 26
- ☐ 2 mls protein-A gel slurry
- ☐ 2 15-ml centrifuge tubes
- ☐ Eppendorf tube
- ☐ 10 mls 1 M Tris, pH 8.0
- ☐ litmus paper
- ☐ 100 mls 0.01 M Tris, pH 8.0
- ☐ 2 mls 0.1 M glycine, pH 3.0
- ☐ 10-ml pipettes
- ☐ 1-ml pipettes
- ☐ test tube rotating device
- ☐ clinical centrifuge

Procedure:

1. Allow the protein A gel slurry to reach room temperature. Transfer two mls of the gel slurry to a centrifuge tube.

2. Centrifuge the gel at $200 \times g$ for 5 minutes to pellet the gel beads. Remove the supernatant with a Pasteur pipette.

3. *Reserve 0.5 ml of the globulin sample in an Eppendorf tube in the freezer for the PAGE analysis.* Transfer 1 to 2 mls of globulin sample to a tube. Adjust the pH of the globulin sample to 8.0 by adding 1.0 M Tris (pH 8.0).

4. Add the pH-adjusted globulin sample to the beads. Incubate for 1 hour at room temperature with gentle rocking or shaking.

5. After 1 hour, centrifuge the beads at $200 \times g$ for 5 minutes. Remove the supernatant (save this until you know whether the antibody was bound by the gel).

6. Wash the beads once with 10 mls of 0.1 M Tris (pH 8.0). Centrifuge at $200 \times g$ for 5 minutes and discard the supernatant.

7. To elute the bound antibody, add 2 mls of 100 mM glycine (pH 3.0) to the gel. Incubate and shake for 15 minutes as in step 4.

8. Centrifuge the gel once more at $200 \times g$ for 5 minutes. Reserve the supernatant containing the purified antibody. Test the antibody supernatant with litmus paper. If necessary, adjust to pH 7.0 using 1 M Tris.

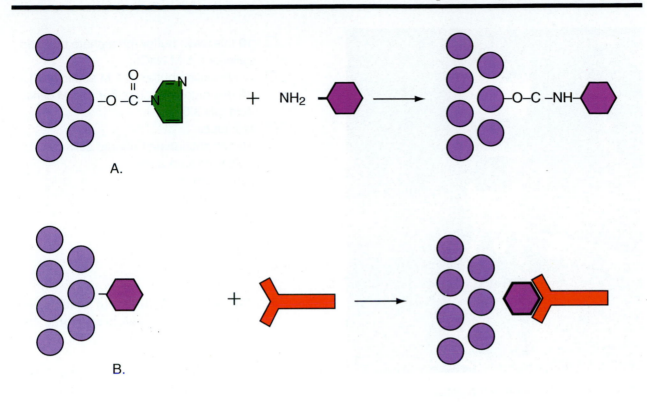

Figure 27.2 **A.** Binding of the protein ligand to the imidocarbonate gel matrix via an N-alkylcarbonate linkage. **B.** Binding of the antibody to the ligand

Part 2: Carbonyldiimidazole-activated Agarose Affinity Purification

A. Binding the Ligand to the Gel

In order to purify an antibody of a particular specificity, the corresponding antigen is used as the ligand. Following binding of the ligand, the gel is treated with ethanolamine to block any remaining active sites.

Materials for Part 2-A:
- ☐ coarse-fritted glass vacuum filter funnel
- ☐ 2 mls CDI-activated agarose (stored as a slurry in acetone)
- ☐ protein antigen solution (10 mg in 4 mls borate buffer)

- ☐ 10 mls borate buffer (0.1 M boric acid + 0.9% NaCl, pH 8.5)
- ☐ small plastic spoon
- ☐ 2 15-ml centrifuge tubes
- ☐ test tube rotating device
- ☐ 10 mls 0.1 M ethanolamine (pH 8.0) or 1.0 M ethanolamine (pH 9.0)
- ☐ clinical centrifuge

Procedure:

1. Remove the acetone from 2 mls of gel slurry by filtering the slurry in a fritted glass funnel with gentle suction. Filter just until the gel no longer drips acetone (fig. 27.3). Do not let the gel dry out completely; it should still appear moist.

2. Quickly wash the gel by adding 10 mls of borate buffer to the filter funnel. Drain the gel again with suction, then scrape it into a centrifuge tube with a small spoon. Add the protein antigen solution to the gel.

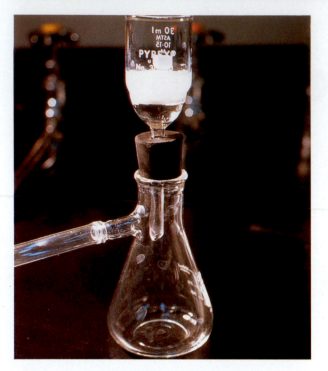

Figure 27.3   Filtration of the gel slurry.

3.   Incubate the gel-protein mixture in the tube for two days. During this time, the tube should be at 4°C on a gently turning rotator.

4.   Let the gel settle in the tube or centrifuge at 200 × g for 5 minutes. Transfer the supernatant to a tube and reserve for measuring the amount of unbound ligand with the Bio-Rad assay in part 3.

5.   Wash the gel in 10 mls of either 1.0 M ethanolamine for 2 to 4 hours or 0.1 M ethanolamine overnight at 4°C.

6.   Centrifuge the gel at 200 × g for 5 minutes. Remove and discard the supernatant. The gel is now ready to be used or stored in water at 4°C.

B.   Affinity Purification

Materials for Part 2-B:
- [ ] Pasteur pipettes and bulb
- [ ] salt cut globulin fraction from exercise 26
- [ ] 10 mls 1 M Tris, pH 8.0
- [ ] Eppendorf tube

- [ ] 10 mls wash buffer (phosphate buffered saline + 0.5 M NaCl)
- [ ] 2 mls elution buffer (0.1 M acetic acid)
- [ ] 10 mls regeneration buffer (0.1 M citric acid, pH 3.0)
- [ ] test tubes
- [ ] 10 mls phosphate buffered saline + 0.05% sodium azide
- [ ] litmus paper
- [ ] 1-ml pipettes
- [ ] 10-ml pipettes
- [ ] clinical centrifuge

Procedure:

1.   Allow the gel slurry to reach room temperature if it has been stored in a refrigerator.

2.   Centrifuge the gel at 200 × g for 5 minutes to pellet the gel. Remove the supernatant with a Pasteur pipette.

3.   Reserve 0.5 ml of the immunoglobulin sample prepared in exercise 26 in an Eppendorf tube in the freezer for use in the next exercise (PAGE). Transfer 1 to 2 mls of the globulin sample to a tube and adjust the pH to 8.0 using 1 M Tris. Add the globulin sample to the gel and incubate for 15 minutes on a rotator, or gently tip the tube by hand to mix. This should be carried out at room temperature.

4.   Centrifuge the gel at 200 × g for 5 minutes. Transfer the supernatant to a tube and save it. Wash the gel twice by adding 5 mls wash buffer and centrifuging at 200 × g for 5 minutes.

5.   To elute the bound antibody, resuspend the gel pellet after the final wash in 2 mls elution buffer. Incubate and stir for 15 minutes as in step 3.

6.   Centrifuge the gel once more at 200 × g for 5 minutes. Reserve the supernatant containing the purified antibody. Test the antibody supernatant with litmus

paper. If necessary, adjust to pH 7.0 using 1 M Tris.

7.   The gel may be reused to purify more of the same antibody if washed in 10 mls of regeneration buffer followed by 10 mls of PBS. If the gel is to be stored for a long period of time, resuspend it in PBS containing 0.05% sodium azide and store at 4°C.

Part 3:   Bio-Rad™ Assay to Determine Ligand Binding Efficiency

The Bio-Rad assay is a dye-binding assay based on the color change of a dye in response to different protein concentrations. The Coomassie Brilliant Blue dye shifts from absorbance at 465 nm to absorbance at 595 nm when binding to protein occurs. By preparing a set of standardized dilutions of the protein used as a ligand, the assay can be used to construct a standard curve of protein concentration versus absorbance. This curve will be accurate, although not entirely linear, over a broad range of protein concentrations. The concentration of ligand remaining in the gel supernatant can then be determined by fitting the absorbance reading of the supernatant to the standard curve and matching that value to the appropriate protein concentration.

If the supernatant protein concentration is so concentrated that it has an absorbance reading off the scale of the standard curve, then you will have to make dilutions of the supernatant until it falls within the curve. Whatever dilutions you make must be taken into account when calculating the concentration of the original supernatant sample. By subtracting the concentration of the supernatant from the concentration of the original ligand solution (10 mg/4 mls) and multiplying by 100, you will be able to calculate the ligand binding efficiency, or percent ligand that bound to the gel.

Materials for Part 3:
- [ ] 25 mls normal saline solution
- [ ] 0.1% protein ligand solution (1 mg/ml) in saline
- [ ] 100 mls Bio-Rad™ protein assay reagent

- [ ] test tubes (about 25)
- [ ] 10-ml pipettes
- [ ] 200 µl micropipettes with tips
- [ ] 1000 µl micropipettes with tips
- [ ] spectrophotometer (visible range)

Procedure:

1.   Prepare ten two-fold dilutions of the standard solution of protein in 0.5-ml tubes of saline.

2.   The protein supernatant may be too concentrated, so also prepare two or three ten-fold dilutions of it in saline.

3.   Do not add the Bio-Rad dye reagent directly to your dilution tubes. Transfer 0.1 ml from each dilution of the standard and the sample to a new, labeled tube. Also place 0.1 mls saline in a tube labeled "blank."

4.   Add 5.0 mls Bio-Rad reagent to each of the new tubes, including the blank. Mix the tubes, then let sit for 5 minutes (or up to one hour).

5.   Use your "blank" to adjust the spectrophotometer to zero absorbance at 595 nm, then measure the absorbance of each tube. Find the dilution of your supernatant sample which best fits within the standard curve range. It may be necessary to make additional dilutions which fall in between the ones you have already made if the ten-fold increment is too large.

6.   Plot the absorbance values of the standard dilutions versus the concentrations (in mg/ml) on linear graph paper. Plot the curve as the actual absorbance reading versus protein concentration rather than as a straight line of best fit. Not all proteins will show an exactly linear re-lationship. Read the concentration of your supernatant sample from the curve. If a dilution of the sample was measured, be sure to multiply

Table 27.1 Absorbance Readings for Standard Dilutions and Sample

sample concentration	absorbance (595 nm)

the concentration you get from the curve by the dilution factor to get the concentration of protein in the original sample.

Key Terms:

affinity chromatography
ligand
equilibrium dialysis

Questions:

1. When the CDI gel was treated with 0.1 M acetic acid in part 2, why was just the bound antibody eluted but not the ligand, which remained coupled to the gel?

2. Is the affinity-purified antibody from the protein-A gel (part 1) pure with respect to antigen specificity? Why or why not?

3. How could you utilize a CDI gel to purify the protein bovine serum albumin (BSA) from whole bovine serum?

Additional Reading:

1. Starkenstein, E. 1910. Biochemistry Z. 24:210.

2. Campbell, D. H., et al. 1951. I. Isolation of antibody by means of a cellulose-protein antigen. Proc. Nat. Acad. Sci. U. S. 37:575.

3. Cuatrecasas, P., et al. 1968. Selective enzyme purification by affinity chromatography. Proc. Nat. Acad. Sci. U. S. 61:636.

4. Lowe, C. R., and P. D. G. Dean. 1974. Affinity Chromatography. New York: Wiley.

5. Johnson, G., and J. S. Garvey. 1977. Improved methods for separation and purification by affinity chromatography. J. Immunol. Meth. 15:29.

6. Bethell, G. S., et al. 1981. Investigation of the activation of cross-linked agarose with carbonylating reagents and the preparation of matrices for affinity chromatography purifications. J. Chromatog. 219:353.

7. Coligan, J. E., et al., eds. 1991. Current Protocols in Immunology. New York: Greene Publishing Associates and Wiley-Interscience.

28 PAGE Analysis of Affinity-Purified Antibody

This procedure will be used to assess the purity of your antibody at each step from salt precipitation of immunoglobulin in exercise 26 to affinity purification in exercise 27. You will run a sample of the original antiserum, a sample of immunoglobulin from the salt cut, and a sample of the affinity purified antibody.

PAGE (Polyacrylamide Gel Electrophoresis) is a common method for obtaining information about purity and molecular weight of proteins. Separated proteins can also be recovered from polyacrylamide gels for further study. Polyacrylamide is the matrix of choice for electrophoresis of proteins due to its high chemical and mechanical stability, but is a highly toxic substance in powdered or concentrated form. Therefore, you will pour gels from a prediluted preparation of acrylamide.

In SDS-PAGE, proteins move through the gel matrix because of a net negative charge, and separate according to molecular weight. The proteins in the samples are treated with SDS and heat denaturation (see exercise 17). Polyacrylamide gels are formed from two monomer solutions, acrylamide and bis-acrylamide, which are polymerized using TEMED as a catalyst and ammonium persulfate as an initiator for the reaction. Most SDS-PAGE gels have two layers. The lower, larger layer is called the separating gel and the small upper layer is called the stacking gel and has a much lower acrylamide concentration. When the protein samples run from the stacking gel into the separating gel, the bands are compacted, giving sharper separation. This type of gel is called a one-dimensional discontinuous gel.

Materials:

- [ ] protein molecular weight standard (high range)
- [ ] separating gel solution (10% acrylamide)
- [ ] stacking gel solution (4% acrylamide)
- [ ] TEMED
- [ ] 10% ammonium persulfate (made within 1-2 days before use)
- [ ] 2X SDS sample buffer
- [ ] 10X TG-SDS electrophoresis buffer
- [ ] beaker
- [ ] gel casting plates for vertical PAGE gels
- [ ] long-needled syringe
- [ ] power supply
- [ ] Eppendorf tubes

A. Running the Gel

1. Assemble the gel casting plates. Make a mark on the gel plates at a level about 3 cms from the top of the plates.

2. Prepare the separating gel solution at a 10% acrylamide concentration. Just before filling the casting apparatus, add the specified amount of TEMED and 10% ammonium persulfate and stir gently to mix. Immediately transfer the solution to the gel casting apparatus using a long-needled syringe. Fill quickly to a level about 2 cms above the mark you made (the gel should shrink as it polymerizes). Carefully overlay the top of the gel with about 1 cm of water—try not to disturb the top of the gel as you do this.

3. Allow the gel to polymerize 45 minutes at room temperature. Meanwhile, prepare the stacking gel except for adding the TEMED. After 45 minutes, pour the water off the polymerized gel.

⚠ *Safety Tips:*

1. **Acrylamide is a neurotoxin. Avoid skin contact and always wear gloves during use. Do not handle it in powder form.**

2. **TEMED is flammable and corrosive. Wear gloves during use and keep it away from flames.**

3. **Ammonium persulfate is a reactive chemical and is corrosive. Wear gloves during use and avoid contact with other chemicals or moisture.**

4. **Never open the lid or place hands inside the electrophoresis chamber while in use.**

5. **Never remove or insert the electrical leads unless the power supply is turned off. Start with the power off and the voltage and current turned all the way down to zero before connecting the leads (red to red and black to black), then turn on and bring voltage and current up slowly to desired level. Reverse this procedure to disconnect the gel. If a gel is disconnected before turning off the power, considerable electrical energy remains in the power unit and can discharge through the sockets even though the unit is turned off.**

6. **Always remove leads one at a time with the other hand free or on a nonconducting surface. Using both hands can create a very dangerous shunt of current across the chest and through the heart if you contact a bare wire.**

---

4. Add the specified amount of TEMED the stacking gel solution. Immediately transfer the solution to the top of the gel to about 3 cm high. Insert a well-forming comb and add enough stacking gel to fill in any spaces. Be careful not to get air bubbles under the teeth of the comb. If this happens, pull the comb out a little then push back in.

5. Allow the stacking gel to polymerize 45 minutes at room temperature, then gently remove the comb and rinse the top of the gel with a little water from a squirt bottle.

6. Dilute the protein samples 1:1 in 2X SDS/sample buffer and place in a boiling water bath for 5 minutes.

7. Load the gel in the electrophoresis unit. Fill the wells with 1X electrophoresis buffer. Add 1X electrophoresis buffer to the lower buffer chambers to cover the bottom of the gel by about 1 cm. Place a small amount of buffer in the upper chamber to check for leaks.

8. Using a syringe, load the protein samples as a thin layer at the bottom of the wells. Rinse the syringe 10 times with water between each sample.

9. Connect the power supply and run at 7.5 milliamps until the tracking dye enters the separating gel. Increase the amperage to 20 milliamps, and run the gel until the tracking dye reaches the bottom of the gel.

10. Disassemble the gel apparatus, and stain the gel.

B.   Staining the Gel

Materials:

- ☐ stain solution (0.25% Coomassie Brilliant Blue R in 50% methanol, 10% acetic acid, 40% water)
- ☐ destaining solution (7% acetic acid, 5% methanol, 88% distilled water)
- ☐ 10% acetic acid

⚠ *Safety Tip:*
Wear gloves to avoid contact with the staining and destaining solutions. These solutions can damage clothing.

Procedure:

1. Submerge the gel in 5 volumes of stain solution from 4 hours to overnight at room temperature with shaking.

2. Pour out the stain solution and submerge the gel in destaining solution. Destain at room temperature with shaking.

3. Change the destaining solution and continue destaining until the bands stand out against a clear background. Make a final wash in 10% acetic acid to re-swell the gel.

4. Gels can either be stored at this point in water or dried for a more permanent record.

Key Terms:

PAGE
polyacrylamide
TEMED
one-dimensional discontinuous gel
separating gel
stacking gel

Questions:

1. What is the purpose of the stacking gel and the separating gel?

2. What happens to antibody molecules when they are subjected to denaturing treatment, and how will they run on the gel?

Additional Reading:

1. Davis, L. G., M. D. Dibner, and J. F. Battey. 1986. Basic Methods in Molecular Biology. New York: Elsevier Science Publishing Co., Inc.

2. Coligan, J. E., et al., eds. 1991. Current Protocols in Immunology. New York: Greene Publishing Associates and Wiley-Interscience.

29 Conjugation of Antibody with Fluorescein

Antibodies can be covalently coupled to a variety of enzymes and fluorochromes for use in immunological detection assays. The following is a simple procedure for coupling fluorochromes to anti-bacterial antibodies for use as a conjugate for direct immunofluorescent testing. First, anti-bacterial antibody is coupled to the fluorescent dye, fluorescein isothiocyanate. Next, the conjugated antibody must be separated from unconjugated antibody and dye molecules by Sephadex™ gel filtration. In the last step, the optimal dilution of the conjugate for use in the direct immunofluorescent assay will be determined.

A. Conjugation of Antibody With Fluorescein

Materials:

- ☐ 2 mg of purified anti-bacterial antibody
- ☐ 1 mg of fluorescein isothiocyanate, isomer I
- ☐ 3 mls carbonate-bicarbonate buffer, pH 8.5
- ☐ 2 15-ml centrifuge tubes
- ☐ aluminum foil
- ☐ 1-ml pipettes
- ☐ clinical centrifuge

⚠ **Safety Tip:**
Wear gloves when handling the fluorescein isothiocyanate. It can cause a hypersensitivity reaction.

Procedure:

Note—part B, step 1 must be done before the lab starts or during the previous exercise.

1. Prepare a solution of 2 mg/ml antibody in 1 ml of carbonate buffer.

2. Dissolve the FITC in carbonate buffer to a concentration of 1 mg/ml, and add to the antibody solution.

3. Wrap the tube in foil and shake gently or rotate continuously for 30 minutes. Meanwhile, prepare the sephadex column in part B.

4. Remove the foil and centrifuge the mixture for 3 minutes at $500 \times g$.

5. Carefully transfer the supernatant to a new tube. Discard the pellet.

B. Sephadex™ Gel Filtration

Gel filtration involves the passage of molecules through a column of neutral polymer "beads" of controlled pore size. Large molecules are not able to penetrate the pores of the beads and pass rapidly around them and through the column bed. Smaller molecules enter the beads through the pores and take longer to make their way through the column. Thus, molecules emerge from the column in *decreasing* order of size. Depending on the pore size of the beads used, gel filtration can be employed to remove small salts from a protein solution, or to purify macromolecules such as serum proteins from a mixture. This method, known as **molecular sieve** filtration, separates molecules on the basis of molecular size alone. Other types of gel filtration involve separation by net charge using ion exchange resins, or separation by binding specificity using protein-A or affinity columns.

You will begin by packing a gel bed of Sephadex beads in a column. You will then filter your conjugate preparation to remove unbound antibody and dye molecules.

Materials:

- ☐ 1 liter phosphate buffered saline (PBS)
- ☐ 3 g Sephadex™ gel (20,000 to 50,000 MW exclusion limit)
- ☐ small flask
- ☐ 15-ml glass column with stopcock
- ☐ column stand and clamp
- ☐ 2 beakers and glass stir rod

Procedure:

1. Prepare a gel slurry by adding 30 mls of PBS to 3 grams of Sephadex in a small flask. Wash the gel beads by letting the beads settle and then removing the PBS layer over the gel. Add more PBS to 30 mls. Repeat the wash procedure twice more. Let the beads swell in 30 mls PBS for 3 hours.

2. Mount the column in a vertical position on the stand. Place a beaker under the column (fig. 29.1).

3. Gently swirl the flask containing the gel to resuspend the beads in the slurry.

4. Slowly pour some of the slurry into the column. Open the stopcock to let the PBS run through. As the PBS drips out, the beads will settle in the column to form a packed gel. *Do not* let the buffer run out below the top surface of the gel pack.

5. Continue adding more slurry as the gel packs. If the top of the gel packs too hard, stir it up into suspension before adding more slurry to prevent uneven packing. The column should contain a volume of 12 to 15 ml. Stop filling the column when the top of the gel bed reaches a point $\frac{1}{2}$ inch below the top. At this point the column could be stored at 4°C with the stopcock closed and 1 inch of PBS on top of the gel.

6. Open the stopcock and let the PBS drain to just the top of the gel bed, then close the stopcock.

7. Gently layer the conjugate sample onto the top of the gel with a Pasteur pipette. Open the stopcock and let the sample just enter the gel. Close the stopcock.

8. Add 2 to 3 mls PBS and let this enter the column.

9. Begin filtration. With the stopcock open, continue adding PBS to the top of the column while the sample runs through. You will see the sample gradually separate into two distinct bands of yellow within the column.

10. When the first band begins to drip out of the column, begin collecting it in a tube. This band should contain the purified conjugate. The second band, containing unbound fluorescein, will remain in the column.

C. Determination of Optimum Dilution for Testing

It is necessary to determine the optimal dilution of the conjugate to use in testing because non-specific staining can occur with concentrated samples.

Materials:

- ☐ cultures of test organism and control organism
- ☐ 1 liter phosphate buffered saline (PBS)
- ☐ 7 microscope slides
- ☐ test tubes
- ☐ 7 petri plates containing filter paper
- ☐ staining jars
- ☐ 95% ethanol
- ☐ buffered glycerol
- ☐ microscope coverslips

Procedure:

1. Prepare two-fold dilutions of the conjugate in PBS through 1:64.

2. Prepare six smears of the organism to be tested on microscope slides, and allow to air dry. Also prepare smears of a control organism to test for nonspecific staining.

> ⚠ **Safety Tip:**
>
> **Use caution when working with the microorganisms. Avoid aerosolization.**

3. To fix the smears, place the slides in 95% ethanol for 1 minute, drain, then dip in PBS. Air-dry the smears.

4. Cover each smear with one of the dilutions of conjugate. Place the slides in petri plates containing a moistened piece of filter paper, two slides per plate. Incubate at room temperature for 15 minutes.

5. Wash the conjugate off the slides with PBS, then place the slides in a jar of PBS for 10 minutes.

6. Blot the slides dry with bibulous paper, then place a drop of buffered glycerol over each smear and cover with a coverslip.

7. Examine the slides under the fluorescent microscope. Look for a dilution which gives easily visible fluorescence of the desired organism, and no nonspecific fluorescence of the control organism.

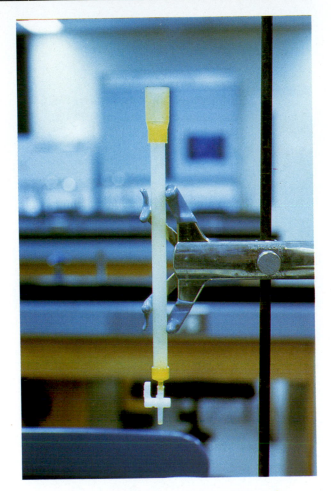

Figure 29.1   Sephadex gel chromatography column.

Key Terms:

> *molecular sieve*
> *ion exchange filtration*
> *protein-A filtration*
> *gel filtration*
> *sephadex beads*

Questions:

1. How could you use sephadex gel filtration to separate the protein components of serum?

Additional Reading:

1. Garvey, J., et al. 1977. Methods in Immunology: A Laboratory Text for Instruction and Research. Reading, Massachusetts: Benjamin/Cummings.

2. Heide, K., and H. G. Schwick. 1978. Salt Fractionation of Immunoglobulins. *In* Handbook of Experimental Immunology, D. M. Weir, ed. 3rd ed. Oxford: Blackwell Scientific Publications.

3. Levy, H. B. and H. A. Sober. 1960. A simple chromatographic method for the preparation of gamma globulin. Proc. Soc. Exp. Biol. Med. 103:250

4. Mishell, B. B., and D. M. Shiigi, eds. 1980. Selected Methods in Cellular Immunology. San Francisco: W. H. Freeman, Co.

30 The Graft Versus Host Reaction in Mice

An **allograft** is a graft of tissue from one member of a species to another member of the same species. For example, human to human kidney transplants are examples of allografts. Transplanting tissue from one mouse strain to another mouse strain is also an allograft. Grafts between different species are called **xenografts**. An example of this would be the transplant of a baboon heart into a human patient. Grafts between genetically identical ("syngeneic") individuals are **isografts**. Isografts can only take place between identical twins in humans, but are easily carried out in inbred mice. Inbred mouse strains are developed by inbreeding for so many generations that the mice become essentially identical as all the unique genes become diluted out. Once such a strain has been developed (like the Balb/c strain), a continual supply of these mice is available as long as the mice are only bred to others of the same strain.

The donated tissue of an allograft will quickly be vascularized in the host and begin to grow. However, without any further treatment the graft will die soon after vascularization because the host's immune system attacks the foreign tissue. This process is termed "allograft rejection." Even a graft from a sibling is recognized as foreign. Isografts, however, are accepted and will grow normally.

Graft rejection is a cell-mediated process, but exhibits immunological "memory" and a primary and secondary response similar to the antibody response. For example, a mouse that receives a skin allograft for the first time will reject the graft in about two weeks. If the same mouse is then given a second skin allograft, the second allograft will be rejected after only a few days to a week. Lymphocytes from a mouse that has rejected one graft can be injected into a normal mouse. If the normal mouse then receives a graft for the first

time, it will exhibit the faster, secondary rejection response. This shows that the response is mediated mainly by lymphocytes. The response can't be transferred in this way with serum.

In human transplant patients, allograft rejection must be suppressed as much as possible. Only a very few patients are lucky enough to have an identical twin as a donor. Most patients must contend with allografts. To minimize the possibility of rejection, several things can be done. First, a donor is found whose tissue is as closely matched to the patient's as possible. The best donor would be a sibling or parent. The donor tissue is matched by tissue-typing techniques such as the MLR assay in exercise 24. Second, the patient's own immune system must be suppressed so that it doesn't attack the graft. This is done by using treatments which kill rapidly proliferating cells, because immune cells that are trying to mount an attack would be proliferating. Examples of such treatments include radiation and cytotoxic drugs, and are fairly toxic to the patient. Newer methods are being explored which involve giving the patient antibodies directed against various antigens involved in the rejection process.

The graft itself may contain some immune cells from the donor, especially a graft of lymphoid tissue like bone marrow. This can pose a problem in seriously immunocompromised patients, such as cancer patients or people with immunodeficiency diseases. In these cases, the immune cells in the donor tissue actually attack the foreign cells of the host. A host with a normal immune system would be able to kill off these immune cells, but the compromised host cannot fend off the attack. This situation is called the "graft versus host reaction (GVHR)," and can be demonstrated in mice by transferring spleen or bone marrow cells from a normal mouse into a mouse whose own immune cells have been destroyed by irradiation.

The reaction can also be demonstrated using neonatal mice that haven't yet developed an effective immune system, or by using F_1 and parental strain mice.

In this exercise, spleen cells from an inbred mouse strain (e.g. Balb/c) are injected into "F_1" mice. "F_1" mice are the progeny of a cross between two inbred parental strains (e.g. Balb/c × C57BL/6). The F_1 progeny do not recognize the parental strain cells as foreign, because they contain the same histocompatibility antigens themselves. However, the parental strain cells will react to the antigens that the F_1 got from the other parental strain. In this example, cells from a Balb/c mouse would react to C57BL/6 antigens in the F_1 mouse, and a graft versus host reaction would begin. The F_1 mice would become sick and eventually die, but an early consequence of the reaction is enlargement of the F_1 host's spleen ("splenomegaly"). In this experiment, you will compare the weight of spleens from mice having the graft versus host reaction to control mice that received same-strain cells. It is important in this type of experiment to use mice that are all the same age (6 to 10 weeks old) and sex.

Materials:

- [ ] 6 or more mice of a pure inbred strain (e.g. C57BL/6)
- [ ] 5 or more F_1 hybrid mice from the above strain crossed to a different strain (e.g. C57BL/6 × DBA/2)
- [ ] mouse jar, anesthetic, and large cotton balls
- [ ] 70% ethanol in a squirt bottle
- [ ] dissecting tray, scissors, and forceps
- [ ] 95% ethanol in a jar
- [ ] sterile petri plate containing a piece of stainless steel mesh
- [ ] 50 mls sterile Hank's Balanced Salt Solution (HBSS)
- [ ] 1 15-ml centrifuge tube
- [ ] small glass test tubes
- [ ] hemocytometer and trypan blue stain
- [ ] sterile 1-ml pipettes
- [ ] sterile 10-ml pipettes
- [ ] sterile Pasteur pipettes and bulb
- [ ] 5 mls heparin solution in saline, 100 USP units/ml
- [ ] 1 ml syringes with 27 gauge needles
- [ ] heat lamp or 100 watt lamp
- [ ] scale for weighing mice and spleens
- [ ] clinical centrifuge

Procedure:

1. Euthanize one parental strain mouse by placing it in a jar or coffee can which contains a couple of large cotton balls soaked in anesthetic. Close the jar tightly for 5 minutes.

2. Wet down the euthanized mouse with 70% ethanol. Sterilize a scissors and forceps by dipping them in 95% ethanol and passing them quickly through the Bunsen burner flame to burn off the ethanol. Pull up the skin over the abdomen with the forceps and cut through the abdomen longitudinally with the scissors. Fold back the abdominal skin and muscle to expose the internal organs.

3. Dip and flame the scissors and forceps again, then locate the spleen. The spleen is the long, flat, reddish organ lying directly under the stomach. Remove the spleen using the forceps (you may need to cut it free from connecting tissues) and place it in the sterile petri plate on the mesh (see fig. 21.3).

4. Add 10 mls of HBSS to the petri plate. Mince the spleen as finely as possible on the screen using sterile flamed scissors. Dip the screen repeatedly into the HBSS to disperse the cells.

5. Transfer the spleen cell suspension to a 15-ml centrifuge tube. Set aside about 0.5 ml in a small tube for counting cells.

6. Centrifuge the spleen cell suspension at $200 \times g$ for 5 minutes. Meanwhile, count the cells you set aside using a hemocytometer and trypan blue stain (see exercise 23 for counting procedure). Calculate the volume of HBSS needed to resuspend the cell pellet to a concentration between 5×10^6 and 5×10^7 cells/ml. You will need to have 5 mls of suspension at the new concentration.

7. After the centrifuge has come to a stop, discard the supernatant and gently resuspend the cell pellet in the volume of HBSS calculated above.

8. Inject the recipient mice (5 parental strain controls and 5 F_1 experimental mice) with 0.5 ml heparin solution (50 USP units) intraperitonealy. This should be done about 15 minutes prior to injecting the mice with the donor spleen cells. The heparin prevents embolisms that can occur if more than 6×10^7 cells are accidentally injected into a mouse.

9. Warm up the mice briefly under a lamp until their tail veins look dilated. Inject each mouse intravenously in a tail vein with 0.5 ml of the donor cell suspension. because intravenous injections are difficult, your instructor will either do the injections for you or assist you in doing them.

10. After one week, euthanize the mice as in step 1 above. Weigh each mouse and record its weight, keeping track of which mouse is which. Remove the spleen from each mouse as in steps 2 and 3 above, keeping track of which spleen came from which mouse. Record the spleen weight next to the body weight of the appropriate mouse. Mice that are suffering from a graft versus host reaction should have enlarged spleens and lower body weights than the control mice.

11. Calculate the mean spleen weight and the mean body weight for the experimental group, then for the control group. Calculate the **spleen index** as shown in the box below.

By convention, a spleen index of equal to or greater than 1.3 is evidence of a graft versus host reaction.

$$\text{spleen index} = \frac{\text{mean spleen weight/ mean body weight of experimental mice}}{\text{mean spleen weight/ mean body weight of control mice}}$$

Key Terms:
allograft
xenograft
isograft
syngeneic
graft rejection
graft versus host reaction

Questions:

1. Why should all the mice be the same age and sex for this experiment?

2. Which cellular antigens are involved in graft rejection?

3. What is the experimental evidence that graft rejection is mediated by cellular rather than humoral immunity?

4. Explain the nature of the primary and secondary responses in graft rejection.

5. What types of treatments do you think would be necessary in order to transplant bone marrow into a leukemia patient?

6. How is an inbred mouse strain developed, and how are these mice useful?

Additional Reading:

1. Golub, E. S. 1987. Immunology: A Synthesis. Sunderland, Massachusetts: Sinauer Assoc. Inc.

2. Coligan, J. E., et al., eds. 1991. Current Protocols in Immunology. Greene Publishing Associates and Wiley-Interscience.

3. Klein, J., and C. L. Chiang. 1976. Ability of H-2 regions to induce graft-vs-host disease. J. Immunol. 117(3):736–740.

4. Marx, J. L. 1987. Histocompatibility restriction explained. Science 235:843

5. Lechler, R. I., et al. 1990. The molecular basis of alloreactivity. Immunol. Today 11(3):83.

1 Appendix 1: List of Materials and Vendors By Experiment Number

A. General Lab Supplies

The following is a list of supplies which are used in a number of exercises, and can be found in most laboratories. All the supplies from this list can be purchased from a general science supplier such as VWR Scientific (see Appendix B for addresses of vendors). The list of vendors provided does not imply endorsement of any particular vendor. Similar products from other vendors may be substituted.

sterile disposable petri plates
sterile graduated centrifuge tubes (conical, 15-ml and 50-ml sizes)
Eppendorf tubes
disposable gloves
automatic pipette tips
plastic squirt bottles
plastic wrap
Pasteur pipettes and bulbs
microscope slides and coverslips
inoculating loops
immersion oil
bibulous paper
lens paper
staining jars
hemocytometers
dissection trays, scissors, and forceps
luer-lock syringes (1-ml, 3-ml, 10-ml)
syringe needles (15, 20, 27 gauge)
vacutainer needles (20 gauge)
sterile lancets
fingertip bandages
alcohol swabs
cotton balls
laboratory glassware (beakers, flasks, test tubes, stir rods, etc.)
pipettes (1, 5, 10 ml) and pipetting bulbs
litmus paper
first aid and safety supplies

B. General Lab Reagents

These reagents are used in several exercises and should be kept on hand. They can be obtained from general suppliers such as VWR scientific, Fisher, Sigma Chemical Co., or Baker.

95% ethanol
methanol
sodium chloride
sodium hydroxide (NaOH) solution for pH adjustment
hydrogen chloride (HCL) solution for pH adjustment
glacial acetic acid
anesthetic (Metafane: Pitman-Moore Inc., or CO_2 gas)
chlorox bleach
phosphate buffered saline (pH 7.2)
normal saline (0.85% NaCl)
Trypan blue dye

Ice is used in several exercises. If an ice machine is not available, ice can be purchased from a grocery store prior to the exercise.

Metafane anesthetic can be obtained from a university or purchased from Pitman-Moor (PM) with a veterinarian's prescription.

C. Equipment

The following is a list of equipment used for the exercises.

Item	Exercise
water baths (37°C, 45°C, 56°C)	several
light microscopes	several
clinical centrifuge (up to 1800 × g or 3000 rpm)	several
high speed centrifuge (optional)	several
magnetic stir plate and bars	several
automatic pipettes (optional)	several
spectrophotometer	7, 27
weighing scale	4, 7, 30
horizontal gel electrophoresis unit	14, 17
vertical PAGE electrophoresis unit	28

Item	Exercise
electrophoresis power supply	14, 17, 28
fluorescent microscope	19, 29
filter sterilizing unit for cell media (optional)	21, 23, 24, 25
laminar flow hood	21
tissue culture microscope	21
cell harvester (optional)	23, 24
scintillation counter (optional)	23, 24
cell culture incubator (CO_2)	21, 23, 24
test tube rotator (optional)	27

D.   Animals

Mice are used for several exercises, and albino rabbits are used for exercise 9. For most exercises, animals may be obtained from a university research animal facility, or even a local breeder or pet store. White mice can be purchased from Carolina Biological Supply Company. Exercises 24 and 30 require mice of a particular strain, so arrangements must be made through a university if these are not available in your facility.

Use of animals in the laboratory requires prior approval by the local animal welfare group. If not available at your facility, arrangements for animal care, euthanasia of rabbits, and disposal of animal carcasses must be arranged with a university or veterinarian.

E.   Specific Supplies for Each Exercise (not listed above)

Exercise	Item	Vendor*
1.	Wright's stain (or Volu-Sol stain)	Sig, VWR, (Log)
	demo. slides	Ca
	mice	
2.	thioglycollate medium	Ba, Sig
	Staphylococcus or *Bacillus* culture	ATCC, Ca
	nutrient agar	Ba, Sig
	nutrient broth	Ba, Sig
	Hank's balanced salt solution	Sig
	Wright's stain (or Volu-Sol stain)	Sig, VWR, (Log)
	mice	

3. gram positive bacterial culture .... ATCC, Ca
    gram negative bacterial culture .... ATCC, Ca
    normal rabbit serum .... PML, Sig
    nutrient agar .... Ba, Sig
    nutrient broth .... Ba, Sig

4. nutrient agar .... Ba, Sig
    nutrient broth .... Ba, Sig
    Serratia marcescens culture .... ATCC, Ca
    mortar and pestles .... VWR
    mouse restrainer .... Fi
    food coloring dyes and heat lamp .... Gr
    mice

5. rabbit blood .... Ca, PML
    cell separation medium .... Ba, Sig
    Wright's stain (or Volu-Sol stain) .... Sig, VWR, (Log)
    heparin (sodium salt) .... Sig
    heparin vacutainer tubes (optional) .... Ba

6. Hank's balanced salt solution .... Sig
    calf serum .... Sig
    whole sheep blood in Alsever's .... Ba, Ca, PML

7. meat from supermarket .... Gr
    mortar and pestles .... VWR
    dialysis tubing and clamps .... VWR
    bovine and porcine serum albumins .... Sig
    Bio-Rad protein assay reagent .... BR

8. *Salmonella* culture .... ATCC, Ca
    nutrient broth .... Ba, Sig
    formaldehyde .... Ba, Sig
    thioglycollate medium .... Ba, Sig
    semi-solid motility medium .... Ba, Dif
    whole sheep blood in Alsever's .... Ba, Ca, PML

9. Freund's adjuvent (complete) .... Pi, Sig
    Freund's adjuvent (incomplete) .... Pi, Sig
    aluminum hydroxide adjuvant .... Pi
    protein antigen (e.g. BSA) .... Sig
    membrane filter unit .... Sig, VWR
    double-hubbed needles .... Ba
    polyethylene tubing .... VWR
    cryotubes .... VWR
    blood or nutrient agar .... Ba, Sig, VWR
    rabbit restrainer .... Fi
    McFarland standards .... PML

10. *Streptococcus pneumoniae* antiserum   Ba, Dif
    normal rabbit serum   PML, Sig
    Streptococcus pneumoniae culture   ATCC, Ca
    Brain Heart Infusion (BHI) broth   Ba
    colored markers   Gr
    mice

11. whole sheep blood in Alsever's   Ba, Ca,PML
    human blood-typing sera (A, B, D)   Ba
    anti-sheep RBC antiserum   Sig
    anti-bacterial antisera   Fi, Sig, VWR
    bacterial antigen   Fi, Sig, VWR
    microtiter plates (round-bottom wells)   Sig, VWR
    50 ml droppers   Ba
    50 ml transfer diluters   Ba
    transfer diluter calibration paper   Ba, Fi
    wax pencil   Gr
    clear package sealing tape   Gr
    cotton swabs or Q-tips   Gr

12. whole sheep blood in Alsever's   Ba, Ca, PML
    tannic acid   Ba, Sig, VWR
    normal rabbit serum   PML, Sig
    protein antigen (e.g. BSA)   Sig
    antiserum (e.g. anti-BSA)   Sig

13. glass tubing for Ascoli   VWR
    clay blocks   Gr
    various antigens and antisera   Sig
    normal rabbit serum   PML, Sig
    agarose   Ba, Sig
    polyethylene glycol 6000 or 8000   Sig
    Coomassie brilliant blue R-250 dye   Fi, Sig, VWR
    pre-cast Ouchterlony gels   Fi, INDX, Pi
    filter paper   VWR
    sodium azide preservative (optional)   Ba, Sig

14. IEP slides, frames, wicks and punches   VWR
    agarose   Ba, Sig
    anti-human serum antiserum   Sig
    IEP markers   Sig
    Tris-barbital buffer   Sig
    acid fuchsin dye   Sig, VWR
    bromophenol blue dye   Sig
    small paint brush   Gr
    pre-cast IEP gels (optional)   INDX, Pi

15.	bovine serum albumin (BSA)	Ca, Sig
	anti-BSA antiserum	Ca, Sig
	glass tubing for Ascoli	VWR
	clay blocks	Gr
	Bio-Rad protein assay reagent	BR
16.	barbital buffer (Veronal)	Sig
	bovine serum albumin (BSA)	Sig
	anti-BSA antibody	Sig
	hemolysin	Ac,Sig
	whole sheep blood in Alsever's	Ba, Ca, PML
	guinea pig complement	Ac, Gib, Sig
17.	NuSieve™ agarose	FMC
	2X SDS sample buffer	Am, Sig, VWR
	Tris-borate buffer	Sig, VWR
	TBE/SDS buffer	Sig, VWR
	transfer buffer	Sig
	protein molecular weight markers	Pi, Sig
	nitrocellulose membrane	Fi, Sig, VWR
	blotting paper	Fi, Sig, VWR
	gelatin	Sig, VWR
	human serum	Sig
	human serum proteins	Sig
	anti-human serum antiserum (rabbit)	Sig
	goat anti-rabbit-IgG-HRPO	Sig, VWR
	4-chloro-1-naphthol substrate tablets	Am, Sig
	glass electrophoresis plates	Sig, VWR
	large sponges	Gr
	glass casserole dishes	Gr
	3% hydrogen peroxide	Gr, VWR
	western blot student kits (optional)	MB
18.	ELISA assay plates	Sig, VWR
	gelatin	Sig, VWR
	anti-BSA antiserum	Sig
	BSA, PSA, HSA antigens	Sig
	Tween 20	Sig, VWR
	Protein-A-HRPO or anti-rabbit-IgG-HRPO	Sig, VWR
	5-aminosalicylic acid substrate tablets	Sig
19.	viral antigen slides	INDX
	FA counterstain	Dif
	viral IFA control sera	Ser
	fluoromount or buffered glycerol	Ba, Dif, Fi
	goat anti-human-IgG-FITC	Sig, VWR
	Whatman #1 filter paper	VWR
	viral IFA kits (optional)	EN, Gu

20. | | |
|---|---|
| meat juice or blood from beef | Gr |
| agarose | Ba, Sig |
| various antisera | Sig |
| various albumin antigens | Sig |
| sodium azide preservative (optional) | Ba, Sig |
| sponge and plastic bag | Gr |

21. | | |
|---|---|
| Freund's adjuvent (complete) | Pi, Sig |
| Freund's adjuvent (incomplete) | Pi, Sig |
| membrane filter unit | Sig, VWR |
| double-hubbed needles | Ba |
| polyethylene tubing | VWR |
| protein antigens (e.g. BSA) | Sig |
| stainless steel mesh (150 mesh) | Ca |
| myeloma cell culture (NS-1 or SP/2) | ATCC |
| RPMI-1640 medium (with glutamine) | Sig |
| fetal bovine serum | Sig |
| antibiotics | Sig |
| RBC lysing buffer | Sig |
| cell culture flasks (25 cm^2) | Sig, VWR |
| cell culture plates (24-well) | Sig, VWR |
| cell culture plates (96-well, flat bottom) | Sig, VWR |
| feeder-conditioned medium | Sig |
| HAT medium supplement | Sig |
| HT medium supplement | Sig |
| PEG 1500 (pre-screened) | Bo |
| gelatin | Sig, VWR |
| goat or rabbit anti-mouse-IgG-HRPO | Sig, VWR |
| control antiserum (e.g. anti-BSA) | Ca, Sig |
| 5-aminosalicylic acid substrate tablets | Sig |
| ELISA assay plates | Sig, VWR |
| sterile gauze | Gr |
| mice | |

22. | | |
|---|---|
| whole sheep blood in Alsever's | Ba, Ca, PML |
| stainless steel mesh (150 mesh) | Ca |
| RPMI-1640 medium (with glutamine) | Sig |
| agarose | Sig |
| DEAE-dextran | Sig |
| guinea pig complement | Ac, Gib, Sig |
| mice | |

23. | | |
|---|---|
| RPMI-1640 medium (with glutamine) | Sig |
| fetal bovine serum | Sig |
| antibiotics | Sig |
| 2-mercaptoethanol | Sig |
| phytohemagglutinin-P | Sig |
| concanavalin-A | Sig |
| pokeweed mitogen | Sig |

	stainless steel mesh (150 mesh)	Ca
	cell culture plates (96-well, round-bottom)	VWR
	^{3}H thymidine (license required)	NEN, Sig
	repeating dispenser (20 ml delivery)	VWR
	absorbent pads and plastic tray	Fi, VWR
	scintillation cocktail	Fi
	glass fiber filter paper	VWR
	scintillation vials (7-ml disposable)	VWR
	mice	
24.	RPMI-1640 medium (with glutamine)	Sig
	fetal bovine serum	Sig
	antibiotics	Sig
	2-mercaptoethanol	Sig
	stainless steel mesh (150 mesh)	Ca
	cell culture plates (96-well, round-bottom)	VWR
	absorbent pads	Fi, VWR
	scintillation cocktail	Fi
	glass fiber filter paper	VWR
	scintillation vials (7-ml disposable)	VWR
	^{3}H thymidine (license required)	NEN, Sig
	mice (two different strains)	
25.	RPMI-1640 medium (with glutamine)	Sig
	bovine serum albumin	Sig
	T-cell antigen-specific antisera	Ac, ATCC
	rabbit complement (low toxicity)	Ac
	stainless steel mesh (150 mesh)	Ca
	nigrosin dye	Sig, VWR
	mice	
26.	ammonium sulfate	Sig, VWR
	dialysis tubing and clamps	VWR
	antiserum	Sig
27.	Protein-A and/or CDI-activated agarose	Pi, Sig, VWR
	protein antigen	Sig
	borate buffer	Sig
	plastic spoon	Gr
	ethanolamine	Sig
	citric acid	Am, Sig
	fritted glass filter funnel	VWR
	Tris	Sig, VWR
	glycine	Sig, VWR
	Bio-Rad protein assay reagent	BR

28.   protein molecular weight markers   Sig
      acrylamide/bisacrylamide solutions   Am, Sig
      TEMED   Am, Sig
      ammonium persulfate capsules   Sig
      pre-cast PAGE gels (optional)   Fi
      2X SDS/sample buffer   Sig, VWR
      10X TG/SDS electrophoresis buffer   Sig, VWR
      Coomassie brilliant blue R-250 dye   Fi, Sig, VWR

29.   Fluorescein isothiocyanate, isomer 1   Sig, VWR
      FA counterstain   Dif
      carbonate-bicarbonate buffer   Pi, Sig, VWR
      Sephadex™ G-25 gel   Sig
      15-ml chromatography columns   BR, Ca, MB
      Whatman #1 filter paper   Sig, VWR
      fluoromount or buffered glycerol   Ba, Dif, Fi
      bacterial cultures   ATCC, Ca
      anti-bacterial antiserum   Dif
      tin foil   Gr

30.   stainless steel mesh (150 mesh)   Ca
      Hank's balanced salt solution   Sig
      heparin (sodium salt)   Sig
      heat lamp   Gr
      mice (parental strain and F1)

      *Vendor's addresses are listed in appendix 2

Appendix 2: Addresses of Commercial Vendors

Ac: Accurate Chemical and Scientific Corporation
300 Shames Drive
Westburg, New York 11590
800-645-6264 or 800-ALL-WEST (San Diego)

Am: Amresco, Inc.
Research Products Group
30175 Solon Industrial Parkway
Solon, Ohio 44139
800-829-2805

ATCC: American Type Culture Collection
12301 Parklawn Drive
Rockville, Maryland 20852
800-638-6597

Ba: Baxter Diagnostics, Inc.
Scientific Products Division
1430 Waukegan Road
McGaw Park, Illinois 60085-6787
800-325-4935 (network sales rep.)

Bo: Boehringer-Mannheim Biochemicals
7941 Castleway Drive
Indianapolis, Indiana 46250
800-262-1640

BR: Bio-Rad Laboratories
1000 Alfred Nobel Drive
Hercules, California 94547
415-724-7000

Ca: Carolina Biological Supply Company
2700 York Road
Burlington, North Carolina 27215
800-334-5551

Dif: Difco Laboratories
P.O. Box 331058
Detroit, Michigan 48232-7058
800-521-0851

EN: Electro-Nucleonics
7101 Riverwood Drive
Columbia, Maryland 21046
800-638-4543

Fi: Fisher Scientific
711 Forbes Avenue
Pittsburgh, Pennsylvania 15219
412-562-8300

FMC: FMC BioProducts
5 Maple Street
Rockland, Maine 04841
800-341-1574

Gr: Grocery Store

Gib: Gibco Laboratories
Life Technologies, Inc. (Western branch)
519 Aldo Avenue
Santa Clara, California 95050
408-988-7611

Gu: Gull Laboratories, Inc.
1011 East 4800 South
Salt Lake City, Utah 84117
800-448-4855

INDX: Integrated Diagnostics, Inc.
P.O. Box 24124
Baltimore, Maryland 21227
800-TEC-INDX

(Log): Logos Scientific, Inc.
700 Sunset Road
Henderson, Nevada 89015
800-821-2495

MB: Modern Biology
P.O. Box 97
Dayton, Indiana 47941-0097
800-733-6544

NEN: NEN Research Products
Du Pont Company
Customer Services
549 Albany Street
Boston, Massachusetts 02118
800-551-2121

Pi: Pierce Chemical Company
        3747 North Meridian Road
        P.O. Box 117
        Rockford, Illinois 61103
            800-874-3723

PM: Pitman-Moore, Inc.
        421 East Hawley Street
        Mundelein, Illinois 60060
            800-525-9480

PML: PML Microbiologicals
        Sacramento, California
            800-628-9509

Ser: Serologicals, Inc.
        Specialty Products
        2550 Windy Hill Road, Suite 219
        Marietta, Georgia 30067
            800-842-9099

Sig: Sigma Chemical Company
        Box 14508
        St. Louis, Missouri 63178
            800-325-3010

VWR: VWR Scientific
        P.O. Box 7900
        San Francisco, California 94120
            415-468-7150

3 Appendix 3: Recipes for Reagents and Materials

1. **Normal Saline (0.85% NaCl)**

   8.5 grams NaCl/liter distilled H_2O

2. **Phosphate-buffered Saline (PBS)**

   10X stock solution, 1 liter
   80 g NaCl
   2 g KCl
   11.5 g $Na_2HPO_4 \cdot 7H_2O$
   2 g KH_2PO_4
   adjust to pH 7.2 to 7.4

   1X working solution
   137 mM NaCl
   2.7 mM KCl
   4.3 mM $Na_2HPO_4 \cdot 7H_2O$
   1.4 mM KH_2PO_4

3. **Trypan Blue Dye**

   Mix trypan blue in saline or PBS to a concentration of 0.25%. Filter sterilize or add sodium azide to 0.02%. Stable for several years at room temperature.

4. **Tris-Barbital Buffer, pH 8.8 (exercise 14)**

   5.778 g Tris base
   2.466 g 5,5-Diethylbarbituric acid (barbital; Veronal)
   9.756 g Sodium 5,5-diethylbarbiturate (barbital sodium; Veronal sodium)
   Add distilled water to 1 liter
   Adjust pH to 8.8.

5. **Bromophenol Blue Dye, 1%**

   Dissolve dye, 10 mg/ml, in distilled water.
   Store in 1-ml aliquots at -20°C.

6. **Veronal-buffered Saline with $MgSO_4$ and $CaCl_2$ (exercise 16)**

   2.875 g 5,5-Diethylbarbituric acid (barbital; Veronal)
   1.875 g Sodium 5,5-diethylbarbiturate (barbital sodium; Veronal sodium)
   0.083 g $CaCl_2$*
   0.238 g $MgCl_2$*
   42.50 g NaCl
   distilled water to 1 liter
   *or 0.1103 g $CaCl_2 . 2H_2O$ and 0.5083 g $MgCl_2 \cdot 6H_2O$

Note—purchase of barbital and barbital sodium requires a controlled substance license. If you do not have such a license, purchase ready-made buffer which is dilute and does not require a license.

7. **Tris-Borate gel Buffer, pH 8.6** (exercise 17)

    10X stock solution, 1 liter
    108 g Tris base
    55 g boric acid
    Add distilled water to 1 liter

8. **Tris-borate-EDTA/SDS Electrophoresis Buffer (TBE/SDS), pH 8.3** (exercise 17)

    10X stock solution, 1 liter
    108 g Tris base
    55 g boric acid
    10 g SDS
    9.3 g $Na_2EDTA \cdot 2H_2O$
    Adjust to pH 8.3
    Add distilled water to 1 liter

9. **Transfer Buffer** (Tris-buffered saline, exercise 17)

    <u>Solution A:</u>   <u>Solution B:</u>
    80 g NaCl   15 g $CaCl_2$
    3.8 g KCl   10 g $MgCl_2$
    2 g Na_2HPO_4 add distilled H_2O to 1 liter
    30 g Tris base
    Add distilled H_2O to 1 liter
    Adjust pH to 7.5
    For 100 mls, add 10 mls solution A to 89 mls distilled water.
    While stirring rapidly, add 1 ml solution B slowly, drop by drop.
    Store at 4°C.

10. **PBS-Tween 20**

    Add Tween 20 to phosphate buffered saline to a concentration of 0.05%
    (0.5 mls Tween 20/liter). Adjust pH to 7.3.

11. **PEG 1500, 50%**

    Melt the sterile PEG at 55°C.
    Add an equal volume of sterile cell culture medium.

12. **2X SDS Sample Buffer** (exercises 17 and 28)

    2.5 ml 0.5 M Tris-HCl, pH 6.8
    4.0 mls 10% SDS
    2.0 mls glycerol

1.0 ml 2-mercaptoethanol
40 mg bromophenol blue
Add distilled water to a final volume of 10 mls (about 0.5 mls)

13. **TG-SDS Electrophoresis Buffer** (exercise 28)

10X stock solution, 1 liter
30.25 g Tris base (0.25 M)
144 g glycine
10 g SDS
distilled water to 1 liter
Do not check the pH of the 10X stock solution.
The pH should be 8.3 when diluted to 1X.

14. **Acrylamide Solutions** (exercise 28)

10% Separating Gel, 30 mls
12.0 mls 30% acrylamide/0.8% bisacrylamide solution
7.5 mls 4X gel buffer
12.4 mls distilled H_2O
0.1 mls 10% ammonium persulfate
*0.02 mls TEMED (add last)

Note—to make other volumes of separating gel, simply multiply the amount of each ingredient proportionately. TEMED must not be added until just before pouring the gel because the gel will polymerize rapidly after adding TEMED.

4% Stacking Gel, 10 mls
1.33 mls 30% acrylamide/0.8% bisacrylamide solution
2.5 mls 4X gel buffer
5.9 mls distilled H_2O
0.025 mls 10% ammonium persulfate
0.01 mls TEMED (add last)

4X Gel Buffer
To 300 mls H_2O add:
91 g Tris base
2 g SDS
Adjust to pH 8.8 with 1 N HCl
Add H_2O to 500 mls

15. **Carbonate-Bicarbonate Buffer (0.5 M, pH 8.5)**
    A.   5.3 g Na_2CO_3
         distilled water to 100 mls
    B.   4.2 g $NaHCO_3$
         distilled water to 100 mls

Add 4.4 mls of solution A to solution B.

Check the pH and adjust if necessary to pH 8.5

16. McFarland Nephelometry Standards

The McFarland standards provide a simple means of standardizing the concentrations of bacterial suspensions visually, without the use of a spectrophotometer or construction of a growth curve. The turbidity of the bacterial suspension is compared to the turbidity of a series of barium sulfate solutions. The barium sulfate solutions correspond to various concentrations of bacteria of the size range of *staphylococcus, streptococcus,* or *enterobacteriaceae*. To a series of ten screw-cap tubes of uniform diameter, add $BaCl_2$ and H_2SO_4 in the proportions listed in the table below. Close the tubes tightly and seal around the cap with parafilm. To use, add a similar volume of the bacterial suspension to the same diameter of test tube. Shake the bacterial suspension and each McFarland tube well before comparing turbidity. To read the tubes, hold the tubes which are being compared against a piece of printed paper and compare its readability through the tubes. The bacterial suspension may be adjusted to a different concentration by diluting saline until the suspension matches the desired standard.

McFarland Scale	1% $BaCl_2$ (ml)	1% H_2SO_4 (ml)	Number Bacteria (value given $\times 10^6$)
1	0.1	9.9	300
2	0.2	9.8	600
3	0.3	9.7	900
4	0.4	9.6	1200
5	0.5	9.5	1500
6	0.6	9.4	1800
7	0.7	9.3	2100
8	0.8	9.2	2400
9	0.9	9.1	2700
10	1.0	9.0	3000

17. **Buffered Glycerol Mounting Medium**

90 mls glycerol + 10 mls phosphate buffered saline (pH 7.3)

4 Appendix 4: Sources of Audiovisual Materials

Slides, filmstrips, and/or videotapes on topics in Immunology are available from the following.

1.   Carolina Biological Supply Company
      2700 York Road
      Burlington, North Carolina 27215
          800-334-5551

2.   International Film Bureau, Inc.
      332 South Michigan Avenue
      Chicago, Illinois 60604-4382
          312-427-4545

3.   Teach America Corporation
      236 East Sixth Avenue
      Tallahassee, Florida 32303
          904-222-6740

4.   Modern Talking Picture Service
      5000 Park Street North
      St. Petersburg, Florida 33709
          813-541-5763

5.   Free loans of audiovisual materials are often available from a state public health laboratory.

5 Appendix 5: Safety Concerns and Use of Animals in the Classroom

There are two areas of special concern which are unique to the immunology laboratory. These are the use of human blood and blood products, and the use of live animals for experimentation. It would be difficult to conduct interesting experiments in immunology without the use of blood or serum, and the use of animals allows study of how the immune system works as a functioning whole. However, special precautions are required when working with human body fluids, and the use of animals in the teaching lab requires careful attention to the needs of the animals and maintenance of a pain-free environment whenever possible. Finally, some immunological reagents are quite hazardous, and must be handled with caution.

A. Use of Human Blood and Blood Products

Human blood products include serum, plasma, "control" sera for diagnostic kits, blood clotting factors, and any other factors derived from human blood. These substances, as well as other internal body fluids from humans, are handled with caution because they have the risk of carrying the Human Immunodeficiency Virus (AIDS) or the Hepatitis B virus. However, as long as the following safety precautions are followed, there is no reason why work with human blood products can not be safely included in the laboratory.

✖ *WARNING:*

1. **Human blood products purchased from immunological supply companies for this class *must* have been tested for HIV and Hepatitis B by the manufacturer.**
2. **If students are using their own blood for an experiment, such as a finger-prick sample, each student *must* handle only his or her own blood for the duration of the experiment. Animal blood is usually a good substitute.**
3. **Never use syringes in any exercise involving human blood products in this laboratory. Syringe needle sticks are one of the most common laboratory accidents.**
4. **Wear gloves and a lab coat at all times when working with human blood products. If there is any potential for aerosolization (such as exercises involving centrifugation of blood), safety goggles must also be worn.**
5. **Dispose of all blood-contaminated materials in a biohazard container for incineration. This container must contain doubled leakproof bags inside a box or disposable plastic container.**

B.   Use of Animals in the Classroom

Recent publicity by animal rights activists has heightened public concern about the use of animals in research and teaching. Both students and researchers alike should be concerned about the welfare of experimental animals, for the sake of generating good experimental data as well as for the humane treatment of the animal. The public is often unaware that any experimental use of animals at universities, whether for research purposes or teaching, is first reviewed by an animal welfare committee composed of scientists, veterinarians, and members of the community. The committee looks for any procedures which have the potential for causing any more than the most minor pain, and may either suggest alternatives to the researcher, or if there is no alternative procedure, offer training to the researcher in methods for minimizing pain by the use of anesthetics. In some cases, the research proposal is rejected by the committee if the potential pain to the animals is deemed unwarranted.

The procedures involving animals which are used in these exercises involve only injections and drawing of blood samples, or humane euthanasia of the animal prior to experimentation. An appropriate anesthetic should be used, such as Metafane (Methoxyflurane: Pitman-Moore Inc.). Carbon dioxide inhalation may also be used for euthanasia. These types of procedures are considered to involve minimal pain to animals, and are appropriate for teaching purposes. However, it must be recognized that pain and/or stress to the animals could occur if the procedures are not followed correctly. In particular, the use of Freund's adjuvent can cause a sore in the rabbit, which certainly must be painful, if not properly administered. It is very important to make certain that *complete* Freund's adjuvant is never used twice in the same animal, and that no more than 0.1 to 0.2 mls of adjuvant mixture is inoculated in any one site. The rabbit should develop only small, subcutaneous lumps that do not necrose or drain. Should a rabbit develop an open sore or appear to be ill (lab animals occasionally come down with illnesses), a veterinarian should be consulted for treatment and administration of an analgesic.

Also, the mice used in exercises 10 and 30 could become sick and die if carelessly left unattended. It is important to monitor these mice daily and promptly euthanize any that are beginning to show signs of illness. A mouse that is becoming ill will often stand alone, and will be lethargic and have rumpled, unkempt fur. Sneezing and nasal or eye secretions may be visible in experiment 10.

C.   Hazardous Reagents

Many chemicals and reagents used in the immunology laboratory are slightly hazardous. The appropriate safety information for handling these reagents is given with each exercise, and usually involves nothing more than wearing gloves and avoiding contact.

Three exercises require the use of particularly hazardous reagents. Exercises 23 and 24, which are similar, use a radioactive chemical. If you will be working directly with the radioactive substance, special training must be given to you by your instructor.

Exercise 23 uses mitogens, some of which are very toxic and are possible teratogens (cause birth defects). These are not as dangerous if you handle them only at the diluted working concentrations suggested in the exercise. Your instructor should prepare the working dilutions from the concentrated stock solutions.

Exercise 28 uses acrylamide, which is a neurotoxin and is particularly hazardous in the dry powder form. It is not quite as hazardous in solution, and requires only that you wear gloves and avoid contact. You should not work with powdered acrylamide if possible, because some manufacturers provide liquid acrylamide. The acrylamide is no longer hazardous once it has polymerized.

6 Appendix 6: Understanding Dilution Problems

The purpose of preparing quantitative dilutions of an unknown sample is to obtain a concentration that can be accurately measured within the parameters of the test system. The concentration found in the analyzed sample is related to the original sample concentration by the reciprocal of the dilution analyzed. This relationship applies to both solutions of soluble chemicals and to biological particles like cells, bacteria, and viruses. The reciprocal of the dilution is called the dilution factor:

$$concentration\ of\ original\ sample = concentration\ of\ analyzed\ dilution \times \frac{1}{dilution}$$

$$= concentration\ of\ analyzed\ dilution \times dilution\ factor$$

Knowing this relationship, the first step in calculating the concentration of an unknown sample is to determine the dilution of the analyzed sample.

Volumetric dilutions:

In all quantitative dilutions of liquid samples, a measured volume x (usually in milliliters) of sample is mixed with a measured volume y of diluent. Thus, the dilution is $\frac{x}{x+y}$.

For example, one milliliter (ml) of sample mixed with 3 milliliters of diluent gives a $\frac{1}{1+3} = \frac{1}{4}$ dilution. Such a dilution is termed "one-to-four" or "one-in-four." One of the the most commonly used dilutions is the ten-fold dilution in which x ml of sample is added to y ml of diluent, where $y = 9x$ ml. Thus: $\frac{x}{x+9x} = \frac{1}{10}$.

Examples of ten-fold dilutions are:

a)   1 ml sample + 9 ml diluent
b)   0.1 ml sample + 0.9 ml diluent
c)   0.5 ml sample + 4.5 ml diluent

Ten-fold dilutions may be expressed as 1/10, 10-1, 1:10, or even 0.10, but exponential expression (10^{-1}) is usually preferred.

Examples of hundred-fold dilutions, where $y = 99x$, are as follows:

a)   1 ml sample + 99 ml diluent
b)   0.1 ml sample + 9.9 ml diluent
c)   0.01 ml sample + 0.99 ml diluent

These are expressed as 1/100, 10-2, or 1:100.

In serological titrations, two-fold dilutions are often used, where $y = x$:

a)   0.5 ml sample + 0.5 ml diluent
b)   1 ml sample + 1 ml diluent

These are expressed as 1/2, or 1:2.

A bottle or tube containing a pre-measured volume of diluent is called a **dilution blank**.

Geometric Serial Dilutions

Because most methods of measurement used in the lab (e.g. colony counts or hemocytometer counts) are accurate only if the sample concentration falls within a narrow range, and because the sample concentration is unknown, a regular geometric series of dilutions must be prepared to insure that at least one dilution will yield a sample that falls within a measurable or countable range. Each dilution step decreases the previous concentration by a constant factor. If x ml of sample are added to y ml of diluent, the first dilution is $\frac{x}{x+y}$. If x ml of the first dilution are now added to y ml of fresh diluent, the second dilution is $\frac{x^2}{x+y^2}$. Then x ml of the second dilution added to y ml of fresh diluent gives the third dilution, $\frac{x^3}{x+y^3}$. This method can be continued indefinitely, with each successive dilution step $\frac{x}{x+y}$ times the preceding dilution. For example:

a)   a ten-fold series: $\frac{1}{10}, \frac{1}{100}, \frac{1}{1000}$ or $10^{-1}, 10^{-2}, 10^{-3}$
b)   a hundred-fold series: $10^{-2}, 10^{-4}, 10^{-6}$
c)   a two-fold series: $\frac{1}{2}, \frac{1}{4}, \frac{1}{8}, \frac{1}{16}, \frac{1}{32}$

The method for obtaining a ten-fold geometric dilution series using 9 ml dilution blanks is illustrated below:

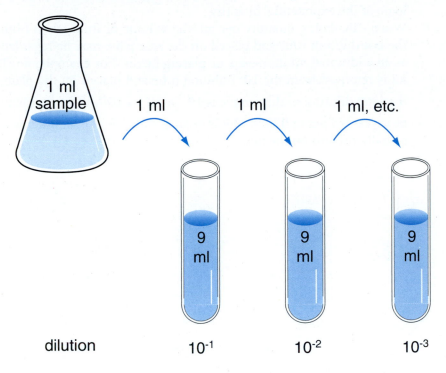

Irregular Dilution Series:

A dilution series may be encountered in which the fractional dilution of each individual step varies irregularly. In this case, the final dilution is simply the product of all the dilution steps. For example, if the following series of dilutions are made, each one from the preceding; $\frac{4}{5}$, $\frac{1}{4}$, $\frac{7}{10}$, and $\frac{3}{8}$, the total dilution of the original sample is $\frac{4}{5} \times \frac{1}{4} \times \frac{7}{10} \times \frac{3}{8} = \frac{84}{1600} = \frac{21}{400}$.

Quantitation:

After calculating the total dilution of a sample, the dilution factor can be determined, and then the concentration. Concentrations are usually expressed as some quantity (e.g. number of cells, mg of a substance) per milliliter, although other volume units may be used. For dilutions involving dispersed particles (e.g. bacterial plate counts) the quantity per ml is termed the "titer." These types of dilutions have several unique features:

a) Accumulated sampling and dilution errors approximate 5%. Therefore, the results of such analyses should be rounded to two significant figures. For example, 748,000 bacteria/ml should be reported as 750,000 bacteria/ml because 748,000 ± 5% could vary from 711,000 to 786,000.

b) Results are usually expressed either in exponential notation, e.g. 750,000 bacteria/ml is written as 7.5×10^5 bacteria/ml, or as the $\log_{10}$ of the exponential quantity.

c) When calculating quantity per ml, the volume of fluid taken from the last dilution tube and placed on the agar plate may be regarded as an additional dilution step, or **plating factor**. For example, if 0.1 ml is removed from the 10^{-3} dilution tube and placed on the plate, the total dilution of the sample is $10^{-3} \times 10^{-1} = 10^{-4}$, if the titer is to be expressed per milliliter. This is because only $^{1}/_{10}$ of a milliliter was actually present on the plate.

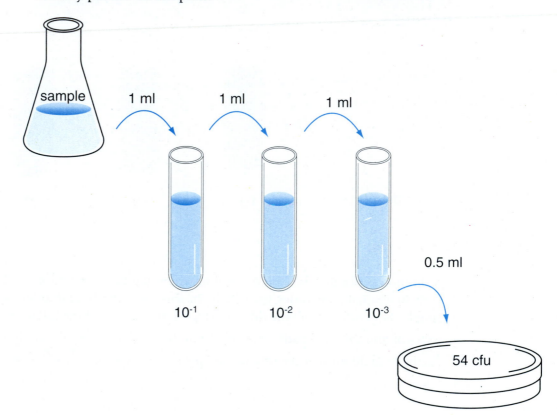

If there are 54 colonies on the plate shown in the above illustration, the concentration of the original sample is calculated as follows:

concentration of original sample = concentration of analyzed dilution × dilution factor

$$= 54 \ colonies \times \frac{1}{total \ dilution}$$

$$= 54 \times \frac{1}{10^{-4}}$$

$$= 54 \times 10^4$$

$$= 5.4 \times 10^5 \ colonies \ per \ ml$$

Another example:

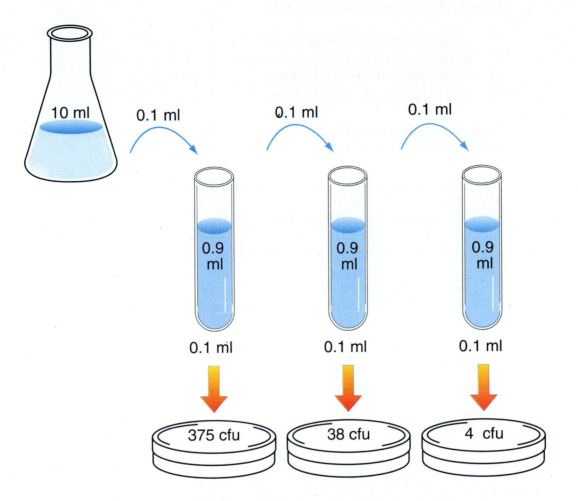

In the above example, the plating factor is $\frac{1}{2}$, because 0.5 ml is $\frac{1}{2}$ of 1 ml.

$$\textbf{\textit{concentration of original sample}} = 54 \text{ colonies} \times \frac{1}{2 \times 10^3}$$

$$= 1.08 \times 10^5$$

$$= 1.1 \times 10^5 \text{ (after rounding)}$$

d)   For colony counts, each dilution should be plated in duplicate. An average of the two counts is then taken for each dilution.

e)   Plates having between 30 and 300 colonies are counted. Colony numbers above this range cannot be counted accurately, and lower numbers are also statistically inaccurate.

Finally, the **total number of particles** in the original sample volume is the concentration/ml times the total volume of the original sample.

PROBLEMS

1. Give the dilution and dilution factor for:

   a) 0.1 ml sample into 99.9 ml diluent
   b) 0.5 ml sample into 2.5 ml diluent
   c) 0.2 ml sample into 0.2 ml diluent
   d) 100 μl sample into 900 μl diluent

2. Diagram a method for obtaining a 1:64 dilution of sample by preparing two-fold serial dilutions and using 0.5-ml dilution blanks.

3. Diagram a method for colony counting at final plate dilutions of

   10^{-3}, 10^{-4}, and 10^{-5}, using 0.9-ml dilution blanks.

4. For each of the following diagrams, determine:

   a) number of bacteria/ml in the original sample
   b) total number of bacteria in the original sample

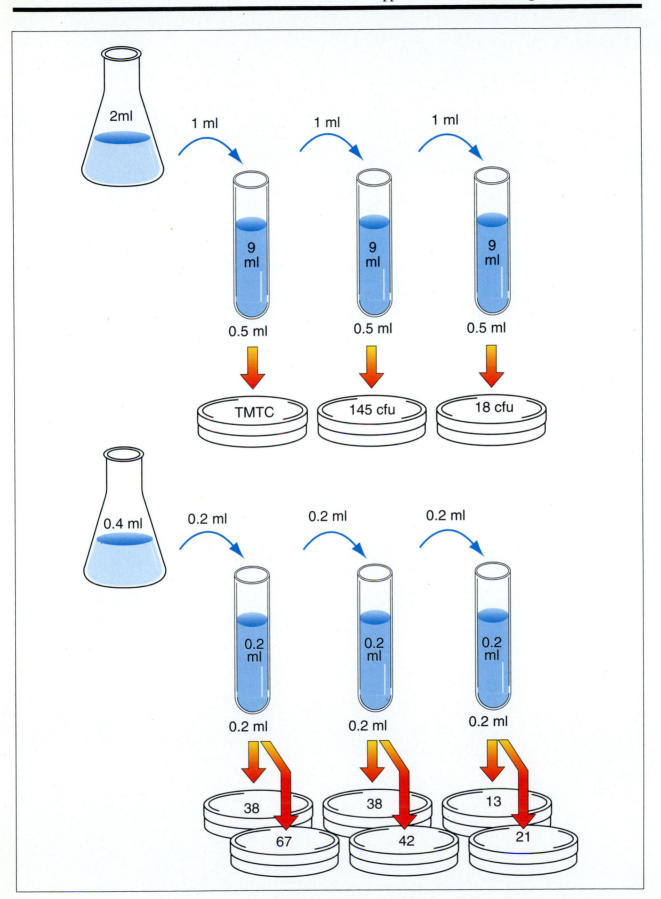

Page numbers followed by f refer to a
figure, and page numbers followed by t
refer to a table.

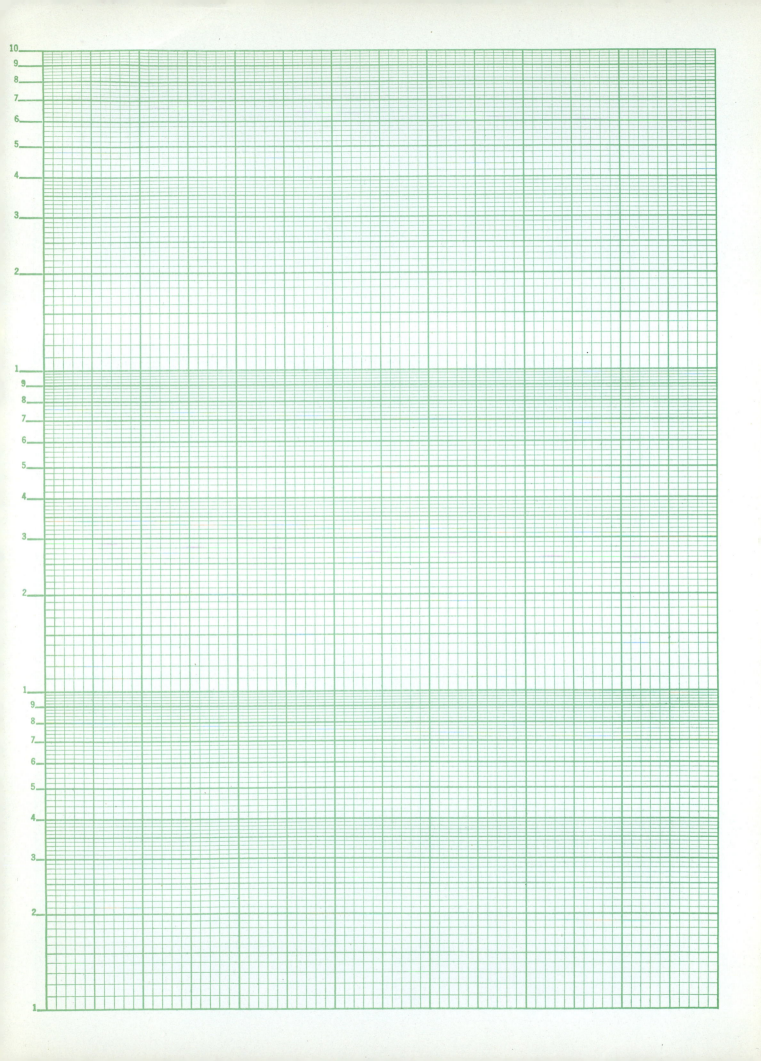